SUSAN CABEZUTTO

In Defeat of Goliath

First published in paperback by
Michael Terence Publishing in 2023
www.mtp.agency

Copyright © 2023 Susan Cabezutto

Susan Cabezutto has asserted the right to be identified
as the author of this work in accordance with the
Copyright, Designs and Patents Act 1988

ISBN 9781800945944

This story is inspired by true life events
though the characters are fictitious and any similarities
to real-life persons are purely coincidental

No part of this publication may be reproduced, stored in a retrieval
system, or transmitted, in any form or by any means, electronic,
mechanical, photocopying, recording or otherwise, without the
prior permission of the publisher

Cover image
Copyright © Kowit Phangkee
www.123rf.com

Cover design
Copyright © 2023 Michael Terence Publishing

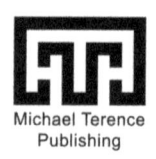

Michael Terence
Publishing

*To those who are so very important in my life.
You know who you are.*

*To anyone who suffers a mental disorder.
I hope, that like Mazy, you find your way
and realise that you are not alone.*

Part One

Prologue

Mazy

The voices, resounding, echoing, are there again. I want them to stop. But instead, they always return. They mock. They sneer. They gloat. *Go away! Leave me alone!* I can't breathe. I pace my room and bite my nails. The skin around them as well. God, how it stings!

I need to check. I need to continue. Don't call me. Don't disturb me, or I'll have to start again.

Family waits. Friends wait. I cannot go. I'm paralysed. The voices won't let me move. They tell me I'm not through yet. They are getting louder. They are demons now.

CHECK, CHECK, CHECK!

How can I *not* obey? I am their slave. I surrender. I give in. They win. They *always* win. I hate myself. I want to be strong. I want to fight them. They grow stronger and I grow weaker. They *know* my weaknesses. All of them. But I'm ready to fight. To struggle to the end. Or I shall be doomed for life.

The thoughts won't go away. More voices invade. There are millions now. They dwell in my mind. They're not invited. But they're there just the same.

ATTACK! ATTACK!

I'm so messed up. I want to hide what I feel. It's getting

more difficult. People must see through me. They can tell something's wrong. The weirdo! Is that what I am? *NO! NO!* It's the mind that's messed up **not me**. I'm not like that. I'm a musician. A singer, song-writer. I want to create. I want to succeed. I'm a pacifist. A spiritual being. But I'm at war. A daily war. I'm a warrior. Not by will but by force.

CHECK, CHECK, CHECK! CONTINUE!

The rituals. Keep the rituals going. Continue. Finish. Feed the compulsions. Feed the obsessions. They'll devour me otherwise. Reassurance. More reassurance. Count. Keep counting. It's not enough. Continue. Two hundred times, three hundred. No more. *Please no more.* My mind will explode.

My belongings are safe. Under lock and key. My room, my sanctuary, all good. Can I breathe now? Are the demons satisfied?

TURN THE DOORKNOB! CHECK! DO IT AGAIN. ROBBERS COULD COME - STRIP YOU OF YOUR SACRED BELONGINGS.

Three hundred and twenty, I count. The doorknob's faulty. It'll fall off, I know. I keep on turning. Clockwise. Anticlockwise. Will robbers come? My fingers ache. Everyone's waiting. They wait for me. I'm always late.

I want the voices to stop. They jeer. They taunt. They never cease. They curse. Are they voices? Are they thoughts? Thoughts I can hear. I'm so confused. I bang my head. I cringe. The searing pain. The blood. The bruise. Immediate swelling.

Explanations now to everyone. The frustration. The limitations. I despair.

And tomorrow it starts all over again.

Chapter 1

Sandy

I've been quiet for too long. Now I just want to put on paper what my voice wants to shout out. It wasn't meant to be a secret. I feared that Mazy could be misunderstood or made fun of. I'm not really trying to make excuses. Judge for yourself. It's hard for children and even adults to understand these problems. I don't blame them. I couldn't understand them myself at the beginning. The reason why Eric and I kept it to ourselves. Kept it quiet, under the mat. Willing 'things' to disappear if we ignored them. Wrong move, now I know.

It was all too much to take in at one go, I guess. New job, new house, new family and then, the cherry on the cake, a newborn. In summary, a whole new life. They all came together. Perhaps not just in that order. But they were suddenly there. Like one big package. One huge, big deal. The love that's there, strong at the roots, helps to see you through, even when the honeymoon happiness is suddenly marred and everything else seems to take over.

OK, so I failed to see the symptoms. To be more accurate did nothing about them. Admitted. Hard to do but, yes, that's the truth. The feeling of guilt is always so overwhelming. Will I ever learn to live with that?

I saw the perfection, the precision applied beyond comprehension. Couldn't fail to notice that. Little fingers on little hands. On a body no more than two years of age. Perhaps less. Yet they mastered those little toys with exuberant discipline and control.

The angel face that bolted like thunder, when those little toys rebelled, and refused to stand tall and aligned.

The surge of lightning, forewarning the explosion of fireworks that followed. Inexplicable and daunting.

A release of a temperament yet to be discovered. A gush of steam that could no longer be restrained. I noticed that, too.

A little head of a child of two and inside that little head, a formidable brain, often fearsome. Inside that brain, a mind so wilful and unexpectedly alarming.

It caught me by surprise the first time. Not the others, as it continued. As Mazy grew, the symptoms grew.

The mood swings. Those terrifying highs and lows. They appeared too, out of the blue. Quite uninvited, without prior warning. Suppressing what little carefree feelings remained. An unsteady helter-skelter of emotions.

The tidiness. Everything so impeccably tidy. Totally unbelievable. Everything in place. In absolute immaculate order. New toys in boxes, just to be admired, just to be displayed. Touched by no hands. Not to be taken out, enjoyed, played with, broken or torn apart. Curse me, if Mazy discovered something out of place. I found it so strange, so confusing.

The hands. They were raving red, nearly always. As if scalded with boiling water. Those frequent visits to the bathroom paved the way to obsessive ones, till the skin took its toll. Papery, dry, almost parched.

Germs. The fear of breeding them, is that what triggered the continuous hand washing?

I saw it all laid out in front of me, like a table dressed for fine dining. Eric argued these were phases. They'd go, just like they'd come. Wisdom that is born of age, would see to that.

I wanted to believe him. It was so much easier to do than accepting what I'd researched. I was pleasantly appeased by Eric, though I was only fooling myself. Denying the obvious.

And I waited for Mazy to grow.

Chapter 2

Mazy

I see the child that was once me. Like a blur. Foggy, fuzzy, misty. I'm still a child at heart. Perhaps because I've been robbed of my childhood. Though through that blur, that fog, that fuzz, the time gets lost. It's hard to let go of the child. And the blur? That still hovers unremorsefully around me, like a bee to the honeycomb.

Reminiscing is so nostalgic. I just don't want to look back but I've got to. My shrink says so. He says I can't move forward, otherwise.

I want to believe him but nothing has worked so far. Try telling my intruders to stop. Tell them they are not invited. They *don't* listen. They *take* no nonsense. They scream in hysteria to a crescendo. Like a chorus in the absolute musical climax. Their dominance and audacity are overpowering. So, I let them believe they are in command. I play along with them. Otherwise, they lose control and explode. With each detonation, they become the supreme authority and I grow small. I cover my ears from the blast. I crouch to the floor. I'm that child again. Confused, scared, terrified, mortified. Hiding in corners.

It's funny, I refer to the voices as if they are persons. But they are demons, instead. Their shadows enormous, greying my innocent mind, in full vulnerability. They punish me for no reason. Fun and play are limited. They tell me my new toys are for show only. How can that be? I want to touch them, feel them and play with them until I grow tired. I don't understand anything.

NO! NO!

They roar, relentlessly. So I stop short in my tracks. And I obey. Such deplorable submission, I cringe in shame, as I recall. Yet I give in. I always surrender in the end. I try to subdue the demons. There is nothing else I can do.

Sometimes they let the child play. But the child has to play their game. I place the toys in a straight line, just as I'm told. All toys perfectly aligned. Like Korean soldiers in a synchronised march.

My little hands comply. I'm really small now. Yet my mind is so powerful it remembers. The thoughts are lodged there, in the rugged mountain plains, the deep secluded valleys, the long dark winding roads of a mind so very complex. They remain dormant but only just. They lie in wait, with unbelievable patience. Ready to pounce on *me* their defenceless prey.

My Mum observes me. She's done it always. She speaks openly to me. Her voice gentle. A soothing lullaby to my aching heart. She thinks by doing that she can get through to me and I can come to my senses. Little does she know there's no stopping the demons. They are ferocious even at the best of times.

I can tell she's worried. More than she dares let on. That makes me uneasy. I want to shout until I'm hoarse. Tell her to bugger off. Don't observe me. Don't be so anxious. It's annoying. I can't take your guilt. I carry too much of a burden already.

'Go away!' I mouth silently.

She's my scapegoat. And I'm a coward. I make her take the blame. I want to shoo my mother away because I can. She's not like the voices. I can't shoo them away. At least she leaves me alone for a while. She avoids the tantrums, the raving and ranting. Lets me calm down. Mum doesn't want to upset me.

I can't tell her what's wrong with me. Where would I begin? I know I get worse as I grow older. Everything is more noticeable now. I try my hardest to hide it. But the evidence is there. Like a merciless traitor, denying nothing, revealing everything.

Chapter 3

Sandy

I feel alone in this battle. I can always run to Eric for support, I know. He'll be there for me and lovingly wave my concerns away. Tell me that Mazy will be fine, and that will give me an instant surge of hope. It tumbles down minutes later when I see that Mazy has a new obsession.

Her bedroom door has to remain shut at all costs. Her bedroom is her sanctuary. All her precious belongings are in there. She must guard them against everything and everyone. Her doorknob has to shine. It needs to be free from persistent germs that can make their way inside. She takes a warm flannel and wipes it clean. Not once, not twice. I lose count of the times. I intervene.

"Stop it, Mazy. What on this earth are you doing? What's going on? Talk to me, Mazy." I am frantic now. I know I can't lose control, for Mazy's sake. Otherwise, she'll clamp up and never speak about these issues.

Her eyes glare at me, as if possessed. Transfixed. I know what I've done. I've interrupted her rituals and she hates me for it. But why? What are these habits she's suddenly acquired? Why does she do this? On account of what?

When Ella is born, Mazy becomes gradually worse. Ella is now waddling around and touching everything. She toddles into the 'sanctuary' and Mazy's face suddenly turns purple.

Ella's sticky fingers mess with her bedside table. She can pull open the drawers. She sees Mazy's toys and wants them. Mazy is right behind us. Her face a picture of misery. I reassure her.

"Mazy, don't worry. This is just a phase Ella is going through. Everything is new to her. She's curious, that's all. You were like her at that age. And Freya too. And you didn't seem to mind, then."

Of course, Mazy was much younger when Freya was born. She was not as obsessed with her bedroom. Aligning toys preoccupied her mind more, at the time. Freya is good-natured and follows Mazy around, like a faithful, little pup. She lets Mazy play with her toys. Mazy doesn't even share hers. Her toys are as new as the first day they were bought. They sit on the shelves. Only touched by dust.

I can't make this out. Maybe I am making a mountain out of a molehill. Forget what I've researched, I say. Symptoms can mean nothing. Not autism, not bipolar, not obsessive-compulsive disorder. They're just tantrums. Stress-related irritability in children is quite common in today's world. Children are spoilt, too. Not like me in my day. That's why they are fastidious, so unbelievably hard to please.

I pull the wool over my eyes. It blinds the reality I refuse to see. I'll do my utmost to keep my family happy. Perhaps that is more than enough.

Stop complicating things, I tell myself crossly. *Let sleeping dogs lie. It's the best way forward.*

But my head tells me one thing and my heart another.

Chapter 4

Mazy

It's suddenly dark. Too dark. I see myself in shadows, midst the darkness. It's the time I have to face up to now. Another phase of my childhood. Why is looking back so hard? Why do shadows overcast my memories? When all I should see is the ordinary family that we were then, and still are.

My parents, Sandy and Eric, my sisters, Freya and Ella. The marvellous upbringing we are given. The undivided attention we enjoy. Couldn't fault anything if I tried. Not much different from any of my friends' families, really. So why the darkness, the obscurity, the dimness, the gloom?

I hit it off well at school to begin with. Even before that, in pre-school too, despite the incongruous situation in my head. Making friends and fitting in is no problem. My mother is secretly relieved, no doubt. I think she crossed autism off her list, there and then.

Her research unveiled how autistic children, generally, find it hard to mix with others and adjust to new environments and circumstances. How they can generalise, I shall never know. Or even call 'normal' what they consider to be normal, 'abnormal' what they think is abnormal. Define normal or abnormal in its wide spectrum, I should ask. I bet they can't.

School work is easy. I can cope well. My photographic memory is an ally. Especially with numbers, dates and formulas.

In Defeat of Goliath

It remains my ally through my school years. They are gratifying and rewarding. Though I don't feel totally fulfilled. There's something missing. Something I yearn for and cannot find. I don't know what I'm looking for, really.

Some horrid kids make fun of me. This throws me off track. Insecurities I am not aware of, kick in. I go into panic mode. I need to breathe deeply but slowly. Otherwise, I shall choke. A red alert signals in my brain. Something else to be vigilant of now. Awful nasty beings who think they can pick on me.

I brewed feelings of hate, of contempt from that day. Little do they know I have demons in my head. Wish they would torment them, instead. Give them a visit. Stay there uninvited. Like they've done to me.

The voices run loose now and the anguish ignites. I become wary. Distrustful, sceptical and disbelieving about everyone and everything. With each step I take, I withdraw more and more into myself. My inner being. It's now me and my intruders. That's more than enough. I cannot welcome anyone else, for fear they will taunt me.

The hurt is too great. I cannot take it. I'm far too sensitive, though I try not to show it. I put on a charade. A ridiculous farce. A masked face that doesn't belong to me, trying to make out that I am strong. I make an effort to 'laugh it off', following Mum's advice. She insists on uncovering the issues that trouble me. I tell her about the horrid kids. That'll keep her at bay. But only for a while, I know.

I feel cornered. At home, the rituals grow wild. The red alert signal is switched on and active twenty-four-seven. I learn to live with washing my hands, again and again. I want to stop but unwavering thoughts invade. I imagine my bedroom overridden with germs. Armies of them. Marching from the doorknob, steadily down the hinges, through an open door, into my bed. My pillow is swarming with them and they keep on reproducing from all corners. Ugly, repulsive, hideous and unsightly, they rally.

I see Ella guiding them in. I feel the bile, stinging and bitter, while it rises from the very pits of my revolting stomach. I want to scream. But I check myself. Otherwise, questions will be asked. And I have no answers to offer. No subtle excuses I can think of, on the spur of the moment.

My skin feels taut and cracks. It's patchy and red. It doesn't look like the skin of a child's hands. More of an adult's. My sleeves are pulled tight and stretched till they are out of shape. I need to cover the evidence. I recoil in disgust. But I do it just the same.

My hands have to be spotless so that I can clean the doorknob of my sanctuary. The door has to be locked, too. Nobody can get in. Not even whilst I'm here. I will not leave my door open. No Ella to toddle in. *No way.* I know Freya won't. But Ella is such a threat. *My threat.*

I keep the key on me all the time. I cannot lose it. I need to check that it's safely sitting in my pocket.

Is anybody else like me? I feel alone in my despair. I dread to be one of a kind and I'm scared, terribly scared.

Chapter 5

Sandy

I feel so sorry for Mazy. I swallow my tears and continue with a heavy heart. It weighs me down, like the heaviest of burdens. I must admit, it's a relief when she's at school. When she's around, her uneasiness is so palpable. Her anxiety is so intense, it consumes my energy. Like a vampire, sucking blood. It leaves me drained of strength. Besides, I cannot forget, I have two other daughters who require my full attention. I need to be fair.

I'm torn between seeking professional advice or giving this matter time. Time heals. It's therapeutic. Time, for Mazy to step into adolescence and gradually change. The words in my diary stare back at me, as I record my observations. I'm sure one day they'll fall on expert hands when I pluck up the courage to accept that Mazy has a problem. At the moment I just can't. Nor can Eric. I'm so sceptical of psychologists or psychiatrists, whatever they are called. Maybe I'll be proved wrong, someday. They just come up with theories and more theories. There is no scientific proof of anything. Just speculations. I'll wait till she's older.

She's already experiencing problems at school. Some wiseacre is picking on her. Others, too, rallying against her. My poor Mazy! I just want to protect her from every harm. From hurtful comments that upset her so. But I cannot wrap her up in a bubble. She just doesn't know how sensitive she is.

Further worries and anxieties are creeping all over her, as a result. Like a slithery snake. Like a coiling root that has a beginning but no end. All I can do is reassure her. Reassurance and more reassurance. I realise I'm falling deeper into the trap. Mazy worries and I offer her reassurance to alleviate her troublesome mind. I comfort her in the only way I feel I can. And the vicious circle spins. If only I could get inside her head. Get to the root of all her dilemmas.

She stands outside the 'sanctuary' again. A sentinel on watch. I want to push her out of the way. Kick the door open and shout at her to STOP. And I do so, one day. I can take no more. Kind words go unheard. Ignored. Disregarded. So I lose control, without thinking. I lash out like crazy and kick the damned door, till my legs ache. The wretched door does not open. It is locked. Mazy has the key.

I grab her tightly to retrieve it and then… I stop short in my tracks. I see her face. Fearful. Distraught. Distressed. And my heart aches with the dull pain of grief. I hug her tightly instead and press her shivering body next to mine. We both weep bitterly. And I express my regret, genuine and sincere, in the hope that she will not hate me. Turn me into her enemy, when all I want to do is help.

I cry again so miserably, later that night when I see Mazy is asleep. I see an angel in peaceful slumber. All frowns vanished. Free. I was a monster today. More monstrous than all the worries, the tangled web of her mind, has ever spun. I wince in shameful pain. And I tell Eric. I shower him with my heartache and drown him in my torment. I observe the sadness in his weary eyes. But he is kind. His words are the solace that relieves my aching soul.

I've done just like Mazy. Sought reassurance when fear and anguish sneaks stealthily through me. Likewise, I will offer her the support and encouragement she requires to climb, so hampered, life's steep journey. Of course, I will. Whether it's right or wrong, I always will.

Chapter 6

Mazy

I fall further into the void. An empty abyss of oblivion. My soul is dead and buried. It wants to resurrect and shine brightly. Erupt from the profound oceans but it lies captive. Enslaved in demons' claws, torn to shreds, till that soul perishes. I want to sleep and wake up from the nightmare. But the nightmare gets more lurid during the day, so I do not want to wake up. I do not want to face the day.

The feeling of abhorrence I never knew, is now incumbent on me. Another intruder is present and in charge. An opportunist that takes advantage of my susceptibility. I don't know how to fight this new trespasser. It doesn't come alone. It's joined by rejection, revulsion and disgust. One big happy family, breeding, blossoming. In perfect harmony with the demons. Together as one. And the load gets denser, more and more oppressive.

I hate everyone now. But most of all, I hate myself. Adolescence is worse than childhood. My self-esteem plummets, just like my weight. I hate my looks. My Mum assures me I am beautiful. She says I have my granddad's eyes. The granddad I never knew. They are the colour of chestnuts, she continues, warm and expressive. Puppy eyes, faithful and loyal, so Freya teases. They hide the greatest story, one day to be told. Thick dark hair in natural waves, frames my face. And on my white skin, just on my right cheek, a beauty spot sits audaciously.

I cringe when I see it. I want to dig my nails into it and scratch it off, till it disappears. I cannot bear it. I want to have claws, like my invaders and shred my skin to pieces, just like they do my soul.

Like the worst of self-harmers, I long to inflict pain on myself. A punishment to relieve my emotional distress. But I cannot do it. I cannot bear the pain. The physical pain.

I've banged my head against the wall often enough, until one day a thread of blood trickles down my nose. I panic like never before. I hyperventilate. Terrified I may have exploded some veins in my head, whilst I banged it forcefully. Even punched the sides of my temples with cupped fists. My aching hands sting and crack, like fragments of glass, from washing them continuously. *That* pain is enough for me. No more or I shall choose to die.

I don't want to go anywhere now. I want to lock myself in my sanctuary, post tedious rituals. Look around me and just enjoy looking. A strange feeling of satisfaction, seeing my precious belongings. All safe. All new. None spoilt. And I breathe serenely, as I rarely do. I do not know what else I can do.

I learn to make excuses. To lie. I become an expert. I learn to say no. But to the wrong people. I only succumb to thoughts and voices. The realisation of *not* standing up for myself is excruciating. I can fool everyone but not myself.

My Mum is more tolerant now. She tries her hardest to understand. So patient, it heats my blood. She'll do anything to see me at peace. Afraid of what the consequences will be when I'm at the edge of the precipice. She's scared I'll crack up. Do something *stupid*, like *kill* myself. Just the word terrorises her. Mum never mentions it, in case I get ideas.

She makes sure she keeps Ella at a reasonable distance. But Ella is a free spirit. She says what she wants, whenever she wants, without measure. It's not what I want to hear. And I crash downhill, right into the abyss, where the dark profundity is infinite.

Chapter 7

Sandy

I try to be discreet. As tactful as can be. I want Freya and Ella to do the same and confront this family matter with the utmost consideration. Offer Mazy the patience and understanding, that I almost failed to give her. Treat her with the extra tender, loving care, I know she needs, for fear she will break up and all that remains are pitiful shards of the person she once was.

And Freya is wonderful. So amazing, it virtually breaks my heart. She is an angel let loose on earth. Her radiance illumines the darkest being. Such positive vitality is so gratifying. I know I can rely on her. She's proved it to me so many times, I almost forget she's just a child. A child so mature, it's uncanny. I cling onto her like a drowning person clutches a straw. Yes, it should be the other way round, but I keep afloat and it's partly thanks to her support.

The words run scarce when I think of Freya. None are good enough. She's like the song, that bridge over troubled waters. The bridge that everyone can cross. Always there, amidst the storm. The strongest of foundations. The hand that everyone will grasp in obscurity. She's so beautiful too, with gorgeously big, hazel eyes that are so communicative. Her undulating, dark brown hair cascades down her back, though she prefers to tie it tightly away from her face. Whichever way she wears it, her hair is divine. Just like everything else about her. And I'm so proud she is my daughter.

But I'm proud of Ella too. She's loveable, high-spirited and popular. Her strong will depicts her. So hard to budge. So hard to bend. She can come down on you like a ton of bricks if she doesn't agree. That's a relief, too. At least you know where you stand with Ella. She's straight and direct. You can tell what she's made of. The good thing is, I know Ella has a heart so vast, its overwhelming. She's a jewel in herself, only this jewel needs strong polishing, I know. *I really know so,* as I look into her hazel eyes, a tinge of green in the sunlight.

Unlike Mazy and Freya, her skin is darker; she has a natural, all-year tan that can be everyone's envy. Ella's hair is naturally dark and curly too. It must be a family signature. The beautiful features in her face are accompanied by a wonderfully slender body, so the chances of turning into an attractive young lady, are practically guaranteed.

Good job, neither Freya nor Ella, let their fabulous looks get to their heads. Quite the contrary.

"Mazy's such an attention-seeker. She just wants your complete attention. Can't you see?"

I do not listen. I try to persuade Ella that she's wrong. Mazy won't listen, either, when it comes to Ella. It's like she's a threatening disease, Mazy has to steer away from. I fear I'm losing the battle again. As long as I don't lose the war, I silently pray.

The uncertainty destroys me. Am I being fair? Am I being suctioned by Mazy, like air to a balloon? I think about it, as I toss and turn, each night in bed. Self-doubt is no longer there when I awake. And I carry on, renewed, recharged. I don't care.

I'll do whatever it takes to protect Mazy. To alleviate her mind and soul. And whoever thinks I'm wrong, can walk in my shoes and pay the toll for resolute attitudes, born of ignorance.

The realisation, too, of being caught in this web of lies and excuses is suddenly so blatant. I keep lying to everyone who asks me about Mazy.

To the family, at reunions. "Where's Mazy?" they well ask. And I flinch in my skin at the thought of saying Mazy's unwell. Or she's been invited to another party. But that's what I say, I'm afraid. Not the truth. I lie instead. I'm getting so good at it, I just can't believe it.

I'm backed by Eric, by Freya. Ella too. And I'm so grateful I could hug them. The truth cannot be told. Not yet. It's too soon. Nobody would understand. Because they don't see what I see. And explanations would be mind-numbing and in vain. They would come to their own conclusions. Their own deadly assumptions and misconceptions. All so very wrong.

Maybe Mazy will change, just as Eric believes. Then nobody needs to know about her intricate mind. Her obsessions, her compulsions, her rituals that gradually bloom, like persistent weeds, determined to push their way through the thickest of asphalts.

To friends and cousins, I tell them Mazy has gone elsewhere. To tennis, perhaps. They find it strange.

"Why doesn't Mazy come with us?" they quiz me wryly. And I cannot tell them Mazy is washing her hands, like a dozen times, in less than one hour. She's cleaning her doorknob, while she counts one hundred times or more. She's in her sanctuary now behind a locked door. And I know she's scanning her room. Every millimetre of it. Scrutinising every nook and cranny, until her eyes come out of their black sockets. Like a lost spacecraft in boundless orbit. Checking that everything's perfect like she left it minutes ago.

And we cannot knock on her door. Interrupt the rituals, because she will start again from scratch. So we wait with incomprehensible patience that nobody else will understand. And we do not tell anyone our secret. Never say why she is hardly ever on time. Why we are all late, as a result. All for fear that she is made fun of. For those who ask are too young. Too immature or ignorant to comprehend what is happening. For fear that Mazy gets worse. For fear she loses it and, in a worst-case scenario, ends up in a mental home. Or dead.

Tell me, what do you do?

Chapter 8

Eric

I could be wrong but I have faith that Mazy will grow out of her 'habits'. I hate to see her in the uncontrollable state she suddenly gets into. Almost unmanageable. More often now, too, I notice.

I keep telling her mother to leave her be. The more attention given to her can be detrimental.

"Just ignore her. Keep Ella away from her," I tell Sandy, again and again. I don't really know if this is the right way to go. But the thought of getting Mazy psychological help is unbearable.

My heart races, like wild horses on a stampede and I cannot take it. My daughter in the hands of shrinks. A guinea pig. A child's brain in an experiment. *No way!* I agree with Sandy. This is our own family affair. For us to know and us alone. For us to deal with. Not to be shared.

When Mazy gets older and if her condition worsens then, I'm sure, we'll take this precarious matter further. But for now, while she's still a baby, *my baby*, I say NO.

Nobody will question, cross-examine, query, enquire or interrogate her like she's some kind of weird being. Confuse her till she blabs out what psychologists want to hear. Then they'll pass their own diagnosis, based on a bunch of words, and my baby's brain will be numbed by lethal medication, that will obscure her will. They'll make a zombie out of her, I know. And *that* will be over my dead body!

I don't expose my feelings. I don't want to upset Sandy, more than she already is. I don't want her to break down. I want us to navigate the ship through the turbulence. Otherwise, we'll all go overboard and sink into this vast ocean of instability.

I fear for Freya and Ella too. I don't want them to miss out on attention. Most importantly, on love, just because we are absorbed, totally sucked up by Mazy's problem. I don't want Sandy to think she's alone in this turmoil. She's got my full support, though I may seem distant, even quiet, at times. I'm only trying to keep composed. Trying my hardest to keep the tempest from blowing up.

But all I really want is for this to stop. I want us all to have peace of mind. Enjoy ourselves as a family. Not be on the edge, almost every time. Dissimulating I'm as calm as can be. Pretending I don't see what's going on. Thinking, wondering, whatever will happen next. How all this, will affect us in the long run.

It's Sandy who observes Mazy and picks up on her changes. I work till late almost always, so I trust her better judgement. Mazy won't speak to me about these issues. She won't open up to anyone. No matter how we try. She's buried her innermost feelings and we can't seem to dig them out.

I take Ella with me, whenever I can, to give Mazy a break. A breather. Some space. I know she needs it. But she must learn to live with Ella too, and all the 'Ellas' she'll come across throughout her life. She must accept her kid sister is part of this family. And *that* will never change. She must understand that she cannot always keep people she doesn't gel with, away from her side. Treat them like an outgrown toy. I want her to be close to her sisters. Know they'll be there for her in adulthood. Like siblings are meant to be.

It scares me not to know where all this is going. I often feel lost. Silently lost. It seems that no matter the hope or the prayer, we always go back to square one. Like the tide that bashes wildly to and fro, but always returns to shore.

Chapter 9

Freya

I feel I'm always in the middle. The middle child. Forever in the midst of Mazy's and Ella's arguments. Often trying hard to comfort Mum, even Dad, when I see his eyes are bleak and dreary, possibly in hushed pain.

I guess I understand Mazy better than anyone. I feel for her. I want her to be outgoing and laugh things off as Ella does. But Ella is a one-off. She's popular, dynamic and vibrant. And *that* you either have or you don't. Just like elegance. Ella the child, the adolescent, the young girl, the adult has always had everyone flocking around her. Everyone laughs with her and not at her. They follow her wherever awaiting her lead.

I'm not like that. Nor is Mazy. We don't have what it takes. I visualise Ella, the child, at the school gates. I picture it now in my mind, just as it was. A second later, she's inundated with friends, gathering around her. Waiting to know what games Ella will suggest they play. And I run behind like a faithful pup, a timid lamb. Hoping that I too can experience a share, however minimal, of that popularity.

Mazy's older. She's not in our school. But if she was, I know she wouldn't follow Ella like I do. She's way too proud. I swallow my pride. I prefer to do that than take the humiliation of being bullied or harassed. If I'm next to Ella, I know that will never happen. She'll defend me at all costs. Like she stands up for others who are picked on. That's one good thing, I must say, on Ella's behalf. She's not egocentric, despite her popularity.

Yet she can't seem to understand Mazy. Ella can't imagine why Mazy is so damned obsessive.

"Why can't she enjoy herself for once?" Ella mutters in sheer disbelief, as she often catches Mazy, totally immersed in ritual. "She's so crazy. She'll go nuts if Mum or Dad don't put a stop to this soon. But they don't want my opinion, do they? No, they are far too concerned that Mazy will get hurt by anything I say or do."

"It's not like that at all, Ella," I try my hardest to convince her. I never do. Ella remains steadfast in her strong beliefs. Mazy is an attention-seeker and everything she does is simply to destroy our family.

"Look at her, Freya, how can you see a different Mazy from me?" Ella retorts angrily, every time I bring up the subject. "Don't you go feeling so sorry for her. She's as selfish as she's always been. Always playing with our toys. We couldn't even step into her room and borrow hers. How often did she frantically punch me out of her room, if she caught me trying to enter behind her back? Can I ever forget those days? You might, but I can't."

Ella, Ella, can't you see Mazy would never behave in this way if she were alright, I ponder almost tearfully. I reflect on moments that are so emotionally painful.

Mum says Ella is so much like her own mother, Grandma Aida. She never believed in mental disorders. Always vowed that you and only you can take control of your own mind. She just sympathised with physical illnesses.

"That's something God has brought unto you. It's his will. But anything to do with the mind is your doing. So only you can do the 'undoing'. Only you can steer the ship or drive a vehicle to its destination if you are at the helm," she'd firmly assert.

Mum repeats those words still. They echo in her mind as we watch Mazy surrender to her compulsions, day in and day out, with such fanaticism it's alarming. I wonder what Grandma Aida would say to that. Surely, she wouldn't be able to disregard Mazy's rituals, as lightly as the sharp words, she always pronounced. Words, like a stab. So agonizingly piercing. Like the ones that Ella so frequently shoots from her mouth, without the slightest bit of empathy.

We all get older. We move on. We turn the pages of our life. We change. Mazy changes too. But her 'habits' don't change. If anything, they get worse. And I speak to her every moment that I can. When the instant seems right for her to listen and be listened to. I tell her my feelings, my fears. I want her to open her eyes and not let life pass her by.

Don't miss the train, Mazy, jump on it. You are made of something special and don't you forget it.

Chapter 10

Ella

I never manage to make her out. Not as a child. Not even as an adult. I try. Maybe I'm too impatient. Maybe cold. Not very empathetic. Call me what you like, but she makes my blood boil.

I can never understand why she stands awkwardly in front of the light switch, for hours. Pretending she's just hovering around, killing time. When in reality she is turning the light switch on and off for the umpteenth time. Checking that the light is off before we go somewhere. I lose count.

What is it with her? Why does she even care about the light? What if we go and leave the damned lights on, so what? What's the problem with a slight increase in our electrical bill? If only I can say it's a waste of energy, she's worried about, but it isn't.

I see Mum motioning to me to leave her alone. Signalling to me with her eyes, her arms in a dissimulated gesture, shooing me away. I learn not to intervene, as otherwise, Mazy starts her rituals all over again. And I know we arrive late, wherever, because of her.

The light switch of every room in the house is not the only thing she checks. She disappears into her room and that's where she lets all hell break loose. She checks and scrutinises her brain away, for no reason I will ever comprehend.

I tell her to get ready early afternoon, so that by the time it's evening, hopefully, she'll be done and we can go anywhere on time, at least. It never happens. And when we arrive, Mum and Dad make all sorts of ridiculous excuses. It's so embarrassing, I vow next time I'll be off on my own. I won't be late. Not ever, because I hate it. I hate making excuses. Excuses that are downright lies. Weren't we religiously taught not to lie?

I know Mum hates lying. She says that's the worst thing we can do. She's always encouraged us to come out open. How ironic now, isn't it? All she does is lie about dear, old Mazy. Too scared that Mazy may have suicidal thoughts. Mazy, Mazy and more Mazy. Our childhood revolves around her, like she's the navel of the earth, in both its left and right hemispheres.

I must be the black sheep of the family. I can't see what they see. No matter how often they explain why Mazy acts the way she does, I just don't see it. All I see is a selfish brat, who has everything. Much more than Freya and I will ever hope to have and yet, she doesn't seem to appreciate anything. Not even the constant attention she receives.

I've never seen her be happy, excited, thrilled. She's numb. I can't stand her. She may be my sister but for me, Freya is the only sister I have. She's the one that stands by me and shares the good and the bad that comes our way.

Mazy does not interact with me. If she did, she'd have so much fun. Just like Freya does. I can honestly say that I don't know Mazy. I really don't. All I experience are her sudden mood swings. Her constant unhappiness. Her anxiety. The tension that hovers continuously, particularly when both of us are present. So I leave before Mazy explodes. Before Mum and

Dad wince in worry. Before Freya starts to calm the situation down. Before everyone blames me rather than Mazy. And I disappear for hours, wondering whatever did I say wrong, this time.

When I return, Mum hugs me and holds me tight. She should be angry but instead, the guilt melts her frustration and she whispers in my ear to be tolerant. I know she keeps our heads above the water as best she can, so I nod reluctantly.

Freya's hand gently grabs my shoulder, in grateful reassurance. I force a smile. I know it won't be long before Mazy and I hit the next iceberg, in full collision.

Chapter 11

Mazy

It's summer. I'm around twelve now. I decide I no longer want to go out and I take shelter at home. I go to school because I have to. There's no way I can get out of that, I'm afraid. I'm glad the term is almost over.

Mum insists that I go to the beach with them. I say *NO*. I'll never set foot on any beach. I hate the sand stuck to saline skin. The feeling of being wet and sticky makes me squirm. My backpack, bikini and towel will get wet and muggy and I fret at the thought.

A deafening voice reverberates through the secret passages of my mind. It's vociferous now, scornful too.

Your precious belongings will be ruined if you touch them with salty fingers. The sand will trickle through. It'll ruin everything. Your backpack will get sodden and when you get home, the dampness will seep through your bedroom walls and damage all. Don't touch anything. Don't go to the beach. DON'T!

The echoes peal and chime, like bells in a belfry, yet they seem as if they're clanging in my ears, and I hold onto whatever's near, to steady myself. I feel I am gyrating at such irrepressible speed, that the world will no longer be able to revolve around its axis, and I will be zoomed off the surface of this earth, like a missile, into infinity.

I'm anguished with the torture. I can't go to the beach. I can't! I can't! The thoughts escalate. My mind becomes a kaleidoscope of flashing lights and shifting images, that reel wildly in all directions and blockade my sanity. Pearls of cold sweat trickle slowly down my forehead and temples. They throb and bang mercilessly. My heart thumps like the deep boom of a bass drum and I just want my head to explode, once and for all. For the sooner this happens, the sooner everything will be over. But it doesn't and I continue in a desperate frenzy like I always do.

I cannot be wet ever. Not even when it rains. I need to dry myself really well. Even at home, after I shower, I've got to dry myself properly, too. I cannot feel damp. My hands cannot feel clammy or the dampness will ruin my belongings. I won't go into my sanctuary until I'm absolutely dry. And another obsession joins the long queue and the burden gets heavier. For me and for all around me. As the obsessions grow, so do the compulsions and the rituals that must quench those compulsions. The intruders come in thousands. I fear I'll go crazy, as they are inflexible and so hard to appease. Their tone is now raucous, like crows at their highest, rasping pitch.

I spend hours, shut in the bathroom. And the family waits. Ella can take no more and bangs strongly on the door.

"Come on Mazy, you've been there for almost two hours. You can't do this to us. It's not fair." Ella's pleas fall on deaf ears. I'm still not satisfied. My mind does not register that I'm now so dry, my flesh is shrivelled. So wrinkled, that my patchy skin tears. Threads of blood gape through, like tiny capillaries that so annoyingly, suddenly float above the surface. It's agony to feel the towel peel the fine layers of skin off my body, like a wrapper from its contents.

I only stop because Mum suddenly interferes. She yells that Dad will take down the door and that this behaviour is unacceptable.

What behaviour is acceptable, then? Did I invite the millions of fiends, that camp freely inside my brain, and do not even pay their dues?

It's too late now. I let them in and they take over. I cannot put a stop to the 'unacceptable behaviour', you all complain about. How can I ever explain what's happening to me, when no one will understand?

They are my family and they claim to know what's going on, though the truth is, they are totally oblivious to my reality. They just huff, sigh, roll their eyes at one another and think that I've already lost it.

Chapter 12

Sandy

How much more can our patience take? I bite the corners of my lower lip, in absolute impotence. I must control myself above all. Mazy can't see me in a state of frenzy, for I am that rock she clutches to, so frantically. A rock called reassurance. It's all I can give her. Each time I shout, she becomes more distant. I don't want to lose her.

When does she start getting worse? Is it when my parents die? Is it when she falls ill and ends up in hospital? When she changes schools, perhaps? Or is it when Eric's mother dies? I'll never know. All I know is that different situations, certainly aggravate her condition, but I can't narrow it down to anything specifically. That much I *do* know.

She never really gets to know my Dad. He dies when Mazy turns one. I try to revive the similarities between them. Those that are more striking. Yet all I deeply perceive are those chestnut eyes, she inherits. The colour of caramel in the sun. The warmth that embraces them, when in shadows. And I wonder if, in his demeanour, there is more of a resemblance. I remember his pessimism. That's what they called it, then. Any trace of a mental disorder was shunned. His anxiety, angst, worries, qualms and fears, if ever there were, went unspoken. Instead, anyone with these traits was considered a pessimist, especially if he showed signs of any 'weird' behaviour. Amazing!

My Mum is different. Kind-hearted and loving, but equally insensitive. She lives in Ella now. They're such a match, it's uncanny. Mazy is older when Mum dies. Around seven. I know it's difficult for her to assimilate death. At any age, it's just so hard to do. So who can blame her for becoming temperamental, irritable and highly strung, at the worst of times?

I see Mazy in that crisp, clinically white hospital bed. So afraid and in so much pain, she finds it hard to remain conscious. The ache is like daggers, so sharp, it scares the living daylights out of us. Doctors talk about bacterial infection, of damned germs. *Shut up,* I want to tell them. *Say no more in front of Mazy or that will generate further her compulsion to wash her hands. To keep clean on all accounts. She'll become a hypochondriac now, can't you see?*

When Mazy moves to higher education, more insecurities lash out, from wherever she has them buried. They suddenly sprout in full bloom. They appear to be evergreens, that never wither away, and are here to stay. Call it a hormonal crisis, if preferred, but they don't help the Mazy that is then born.

And when Eric's mother dies? Mazy's so impacted that she can't overcome it. She asks questions to which there are no answers. Remember the good memories lived, Mazy, I try to tell her. No balm, this time, to soothe the hurt. Only time can see to that.

Whatever the circumstances, it's still unclear how Mazy worsens. All I know is that I become a referee, in life's most complicated match. And I don't know how many more yellow or red flags, I can wave at the player's faces, to make them recognise foul play. Get them to follow the rules, for ease of living, not existing. For fear that the dreaded day will come, when all this blows seriously, out of proportion.

Chapter 13

Mazy

I walk out of school. A lanky student in aimless stride. With aimless goals. A promise of an aimless future. It darkens my horizons and I cannot focus. But with every step, I know I'm closer to my mission. A mission I've been contemplating, long and through. It does not scare me. Only then, can I end this torment.

The suicidal thoughts that haunt me, dwell in my head for quite some time. Invaders of a different kind. And I find myself in full strategy. Conniving, scheming, calculating in sheer silence, every possible outcome. How would I do it? What would I use to end it all? Where would I go to see it through? At home? Elsewhere?

I'm at my doorstep and I don't know how I've arrived. So lost in thought, a car could've run me over. No need to lift a finger then, to end my anguish.

In front of me is Freya. Her angel face and angel eyes pierce through mine, with such penetrating force, it's like she can read my most innate thoughts. They are like a show of the cross, against the dark evil will of any devil. And she stays with me for the rest of the day, trying her utmost to generate interesting conversation. As if she has a sixth sense, that is telling her, *hey keep watch over Mazy, she's going to do something really appalling.*

She knows I won't disappear into my sanctuary, until late. The everlasting rituals, keep me from doing so. Besides, everyone's around now and it's so awkward to carry them out, without being observed. So Freya sits with me and we watch a movie before dinner. I appreciate, wholeheartedly, what she's doing. I enjoy her company.

It won't be long before Ella claims her attention and I will stay on my own, as always. I'm sure Mum will step in then, and try to chat me up. Try to psycho-analyse me, no doubt.

Cut the small talk, I want to retort. *I'm not crazy or some kind of lunatic. I know exactly what I'm doing. It's the thoughts, the voices, the demons, or call them what you want, in my mind, I can't control.*

The film continues and whilst surreal beasts fight, in full fury, in unknown planets not yet discovered, my thoughts are on my silent plan. I can't believe this motivates me. And I continue to deal and wheel the perfect plot like it was the perfect crime.

Would I use a knife to end it all? Could I possibly thrust its razor-sharp blade inside me? Slit my wrists open? How about a rope? Could I throw a rope over some wooden beam in the ceiling of some place? Knot it around my neck, like I've seen in movies, so many times. They make it look so easy. But is it? The last thing I want to do, if I attempt suicide, is fail miserably.

Do I have what it takes? How do people do it? Are they half-drunk, half-drugged? They must be. I guess it's so much easier to throw yourself off a cliff. Or through an open window of a twelfth floor. But it's so ironic. *I'm* so ironic. I hate physical pain. I can't take anymore. How could I ever go ahead with suicide? Perhaps a lethal overdose is even easier. Would I fall asleep with no pain? The thoughts are one thing, the reality another.

I steer my vision towards my Mum, busily preparing Ella's favourite. Little does she know that what she suspects, is in my mind already and in process. I cower with sudden, unexpected sadness, in anticipation of the terrible pain I will inflict on loved ones.

And I force my thoughts back to the beasts, this time not the ones in my mind but those incredulous creatures in the Sci-Fi movie, now conquerors of new kingdoms, hidden in the vast orbits of the cosmos.

I feel the tears well in my eyes. For now, my plans are shattered.

Chapter 14

Freya

I mention it to Mum. I fear for Mazy. She's more withdrawn than she's ever been. Even at school. She hangs around with a couple of friends but I can't say they are a good influence either. Or vice-versa, in all fairness. Mazy is too lonely, but she does not want my company outside the house. So we don't go anywhere together. I suggest we join a club, any club but she always says *no way*.

I have this uneasy feeling, that she might end her life one day. I have visions, deadly visions that impair my will. I see her on the top floor of a building, climbing onto the waist-high wall of the outdoor landing. Her steps falter, as she prepares for her final countdown. Stealing a look down the many metres to the ground and steadying herself, lest she falls before she's ready. Then the inevitable.

She closes her eyes and slowly forces her body forward to the very edge. And I scream DON'T! But the words are silent and it's too late, for she is in full flight. With arms outstretched, she glides down like a graceful swan, only the sight is devastating. And I don't want to stare at the rag doll strewn below, for that is what she'll be, a broken doll, with limbs unrecognisably contorted. Blood will carpet the ground beneath her and the feeling of doom will hit me with its strongest blow.

Mum says she will take action. She doesn't want to wait much longer. We don't see Mazy getting any better. In the end, she'll need to seek psychological help, as much as she's been avoiding this. Who knows, I tell her, it may be for the best.

All this business really upsets me. Now it's just the two of us most of them time, Ella and I. There are people, who don't even know or remember I have an older sister. Who can blame them? They never see the three of us together anymore.

And I miss Mazy so. I pray nothing bad happens to her. But what I see scares me. I try to speak to her like many a time before when at least she seemed to listen. But she just waves me away now, like a pestering fly, when I hit the subject. She'll speak of other things, though. But the wall is always there between us. And no wrecking ball can crush it down to rubble.

There must be something that Mazy can enjoy. Something that can take her mind off obstacles. Keep her busy and entertained. Give her some comfort in her critical moments.

I see she's got her headphones on. Is she listening to music? Or pretending to? Does she put them on to keep everyone from speaking to her?

I must admit Mazy is exasperating. Ella is right to some extent. I won't confess this though, otherwise, that will give Ella reason enough to become more confrontational. And *that* won't help any of us.

I'll just have to be as tolerant as can be and hope that Ella follows suit. The storm or call it the war that is slowly fermenting cannot blast, because the consequences, I predict, will be utterly demolishing.

Chapter 15

Mazy

I'll take drugs then. Start smoking weed. Maybe even something stronger. I need something. I'll move in those circles. Turn to alcohol, perhaps. Something. If I can't commit suicide, then what's next? And my mind races once again, in search of that miracle that doesn't exist. For deep in the furthest crevices of my heart, I know there isn't one. Yet I enjoy scheming and dreaming. It seems to give me an incentive. Pity I need an incentive of that type.

I should be thinking of my future instead. Dreaming about what I could be. But my mind is vague, too foggy to focus on anything good. For I know the demons won't allow it. They tell me I cannot succeed. That I have no future. I don't even know what I like anymore. And if I *do* like something, I quickly erase it from my mind for fear they'll know and jeer.

Then the mocking starts and I hear them say: *You - have you just seen yourself? Do you think you can be a lawyer, a teacher, a nurse? You don't have what it takes. You're a loser. You'll never succeed. So why even bother doing well at school?*

I sigh, a deep sigh that exhales so much negative energy, I'm glad I'm on my own with my headphones on, listening to Kurt Corbain's 'About a Girl'. *He* would know what I'm talking about if he were still around. He seems to sing my life like he was living it. 'Come as you are' follows and my fingers, instinctively, tap away to the music of his guitar.

And I realise, suddenly, that my fingers rebel against the voices in my head, and they will not be coerced by demons. Because they sense the music, as it runs through icy veins, and the ice gradually melts. It gives way to fire, a burning sensation, as they listen to Kurt's voice, in splendorous chant.

Next, my feet do the tapping. There's no control over them. They're free. And when they listen to Blink 182, they become wild, ecstatically feral, almost. They don't belong to a body, stuck to a head, where inside that head lives a mind so dominant, it holds every limb to its mercy. They are in full rebellion now. They are mutinying. They don't want to be deprived. They're on a high. In full elation. Better than any elation from any drug.

The demons can't be caught off guard. They take up their post in full command. Wary that something different is happening. So they file the ranks without question or delay. But Blink 182 stands no nonsense. It drains their voices and mutes them. So fingers continue tapping to the magical beat of bass guitars and drums. Feet continue tapping to the strumming of lead guitars and the marvellous voices of lead singers, making a mockery of demons' voices.

For hours I sit, surprisingly serene, listening with what little strength remains in me. Feeling the music flowing, slowly, through every nook of my body. I tingle, even quiver. I'm aware my hairs are on end. I'm not terrified, for once, just extremely and unbelievably tranquil.

And the balm I've been searching for is unexpectedly here, soothing me in mind and soul, like never before.

Chapter 16

Sandy

I so wish Mazy would find herself a hobby. Something to keep her occupied. There are millions of things I know she'd love to do if she wasn't chained, imprisoned in the cell of her mind. She has no free will. Despite our long chats, I am fully aware that as much as she may try, she's totally restrained. Unable to liberate herself from the shackles that bind her, in mind and soul.

I know Mazy is so talented. I'm sure she'd be brilliant at whatever she chose to do. But it breaks my heart to see her completely inhibited. Cornered like a rat, even at the best of times.

I tell her to take up some sport. Any. She nods, possibly to shut me up. I know she doesn't like where this conversation is going, so she wants to end it, no matter what.

"How about the arts and crafts?" I continue slowly, trying to see if there is a spark in her eyes. Anything that may give me an indication of hope. Hope that she will get a little joy out of something. Hope that she will meet new friends with whom to socialise, in some way or other. But hope doesn't seem to be there. It does not live in her and consequently cannot be professed.

"Books? Interested in reading? Here are some authors you may enjoy." Again, the vagueness in her response, tells me to stop. Not to push further. And all I can do is cringe in fretful despair. A despair inside of me, I don't want her to perceive.

Freya worries terribly over Mazy. She confesses her fears. I don't admit to her that what she dreads, I dread too, only threefold. Suicide is my worst fear. It keeps me awake, tossing and turning. Giving me nightmares, even during the day. I cannot let this situation get the better of me. For Mazy's sake, I know I must act - and fast. Who am I trying to fool? Even Freya can see Mazy isn't getting any better. If anything that drastic should happen to Mazy, I know my life would end with hers. I must seek professional advice. I reckon there's no other way forward.

I may be doing Mazy no good just by offering her reassurance when she seems to lose it. I speak to her gently and it calms her down, if only for a short while. I assure her that everything will be alright. Her belongings, her sanctuary, they're all good, I almost whisper in her ear. Her life, her future, they'll be wonderful, I promise her. Nobody will enter her sanctuary. The door will always be locked. Only she has the key. There are no others. Nobody will touch anything, not Ella, not anyone. No dampness, no rain will damage her room, I desperately reiterate. I lose count of the times I have to repeat the same words and phrases, over and over, till her mind registers that everything is fine. Nothing is that shockingly bad.

And if I see a ray of hope in her eyes, I feel I've conquered the world. I'm so relieved to see her relieved, that I don't care if we're falling further and further into the trap. If I can see a smile on her face, even if it's a forced one, I know I am winning.

We are winning. And I continue in a daily battle. Determined to win the war.

Chapter 17

Mazy

The demons retaliate. They seek revenge. Like they always do. Only this time, it's worse, because they are livid. They are beside themselves with rage. Their stomping reverberates through the corners of my mind and I imagine they've developed into belligerent giants. Aggressive, fuming with uncontrollable wrath. They'll stop at nothing now, just because they did not win the last battle. Their voices were drowned and the music conquered. And it felt so good to have the music invade my inner being. It consumed me entirely, in body and soul. They knocked the demons unconscious. One to me - for once!

Nothing like this has ever happened to me before. I felt a serenity that made my spirit float. That moment was one of a kind. I felt alive and energised but completely calm at the same time. Like I was drifting above the clouds, into eternity. Transported to a whole new world. A world I thoroughly enjoyed, and want more of. Is this what I've been searching for all this time? Is this what I need to fill the empty void inside of me?

I've never given music much thought before. Maybe because I never really listened hard enough. But I listened yesterday. I listened really hard and I felt it palpitating through each fibre of my body, much faster than any heartbeat. And it felt so wonderfully wonderful. All the very senses in me were tuned to the rhythm of each beat, each tempo. And I found I could breathe freely, without choking.

Is it true I ignored the demons? *I couldn't possibly!* Did I actually do so? I knew they were screaming at me to take my headphones off and turn the music down. But my fingers and feet did not listen. They almost made me stand up to dance to the marvellous rhythm, that travelled so wildly through my veins.

I don't think any drug could have taken me to this euphoric level. And I crave more. I want more ecstatic moments in my life. Once you get a piece of the cake, you have to take a bite and savour the taste. A slow, long-lasting mouthful to relish the instant. Engrave it in the mind. Use it as a weapon to hit back. For until now, I've been defenceless.

And music becomes my ally. But the demons in my head attack me now, without remorse. They revel in joy, as they start with a hissing undertone.

Your hands are clammy, sticky, filthy. You can't put your headphones on. You can't listen to the music because you have to shower, dry yourself thoroughly and that will take hours. Then you have to study but you can't enter your sanctuary because the door knob isn't clean. What about the key, is it in your pocket? CHECK! CHECK!

The demons do not murmur any longer. They yell now with all their might. My goodness! What is it they bawl so vehemently about? It deafens me intensely and I cover my ears or they will burst, I'm sure.

DO YOU THINK YOU ARE FREE TO DO WHAT YOU WANT, WHEN YOU WANT, HOW YOU WANT? YOU ARE CONDEMNED FOR LIFE AND DON'T YOU FORGET IT.

And my heart sinks, yet again, to the greatest depths of despair. I know all this will bring grave consequences, so I shudder in my skin, at the impending torment ahead.

My headphones suddenly become remote, unreachable. The music is totally inaccessible.

Chapter 18

Eric

Sandy is under a lot of pressure lately. I feel for her. In the end, *she'll* be the one to have a nervous breakdown and not Mazy, if she's not careful. She's so confused about which way to go. I'm partly to blame for her not having taken action already. She's aware of how dead against it I am. Though I must agree, Mazy isn't making any progress. She doesn't snap out of those damned rituals I discreetly catch her doing. I hide the moment I see her, to save her the humiliation. I know how much she hates being observed.

I hate the fact we can't seem to be together as a family anymore, all of us, I mean. Whenever we are all together, a brawl of the worst kind breaks out between Ella and Mazy. They don't stop shouting blue murder at each other, until Sandy or I intervene. And then each goes off in a huff, leaving us alone with poor Freya, not knowing which side to take.

Ella will show Mazy up, no matter how much we tell her to be tactful. She'll comment on her parched hands. She'll bring up the rituals she too has caught Mazy in the midst of, more than once. That will mortify Mazy and her measured anger twists, uncontrollably, into a frightful outburst.

It really saddens me. I thought their stupid bickering would end as they grew older, but it's just not happening. It scares me to think they could turn to their hands one day. It would break my heart to witness that.

I guess we are all tired of their continuous insolence; the offensive language that they profess to each other is totally uncalled for and unacceptable. Mostly we are all tired of mediating between the two. We explain firmly the consequences of such appalling behaviour, but they don't listen and shrug off our words, listlessly. Like they think something drastic would never happen. Their fury blinds them. Their pride too.

I end up at work even at weekends. I'm not really trying to escape from the web that has gradually spun at home. There's work to be done and I have to be there. I feel I'm leaving Sandy with the brunt of it all, though. She doesn't really complain much or even nag at me. Only when she needs to let off some steam or feels somewhat vulnerable, does she turn to me for reassurance.

I know Sandy does not want to create divisions by keeping Ella at a considerable 'distance', to give Mazy both the space and the time alone she requires. But no doubt, that is what's happening and I don't exactly approve. I realise it avoids arguments and confrontations but I don't want to see our family torn apart, no matter in which way.

It's a real chore to be completely fair to everyone under these circumstances. I really don't know how we face the day, when there's no knowing what will suddenly blast in our faces. It's as if we live each day holding hand grenades. Ridiculously hoping that they won't detonate, yet conscious that at any moment, they undoubtedly will.

Chapter 19

Mazy

The impending torment I so dreaded, devours me with inexplicable vigour. A tsunami of the worst kind. A tidal wave towering above me with the mightiest of force. And I know it will not pass rapidly by. It's here to stay; to show me who's the grand boss and who's the subordinate.

They are torturing me now, as only *they* know how. Confusing my wits until all I can think, is that I've murdered somebody. Just like that! Just as simple! Those treacherous voices keep hounding me. Jarring my mind, until it reels in instant panic.

You criminal, you! Do you know what you are? A criminal, a murderer, a killer. Name it what you like, but that's what you've become.

A sudden fear seizes my senses from scalp to toe. Such a cold terror that can only be compared to death itself. The feeling of doom. And I am automatically transformed into what they want me to be. A useless being. Incapable of standing up to myself and retorting to the demons, as I know I should.

How on earth can I be a criminal of any kind when I'm at school all day? Then I return home and hardly ever go out. When I do, it's never on my own, you suckers!

That's what I *should* retort. But instead, I shrink further and further into myself. The little girl is back again. Squatting in a corner with the palms of her hands opened wide and covering her ears. Though sadly, nothing works. Because nothing, absolutely nothing, stops the demons from antagonising me, as they seek their revenge.

They gloat now, rejoicing triumphantly that yet again they've won. I won a battle but they win the war, like always. How could I have been so stupid as to defy them? Did I think the wonderful sound of the music pumping through my veins could be my ally? And that together we could conquer the tireless monsters that dwell in my mind. How could I even think of it? How naive! How very, very innocent. An innocence so vulnerable, no wonder they chose me.

My mind is telling me all the crazy things I don't want to hear. It says I killed someone when we went on that school trip. That stupid trip that had me sunburnt for weeks. I should have followed my instincts and not gone, knowing how much I hate being wet. But I gave myself a chance. A chance to maybe enjoy myself for once with the few 'friends' I feel at ease among.

Not that I've divulged anything that goes on in my mind to any of them. They can continue thinking I'm some kind of weirdo. Eccentric perhaps. Just because I don't open up to anyone when they fire their endless questions at me. And I just shrug them off, just like I do to my parents. Till I see them shrug me off too, and give up.

My panic mode does not switch itself off. And I fall into bitter hopelessness. I need reassurance badly like junkies need their fix. The voices keep retorting to my incredulous questions.

How could I have killed on that trip? How, where, when, who? I alarmingly ask. And they respond in haste and with such steadfast conviction that I squirm and just want to throw up. The acid from the bile makes its way through my thorax, stinging my throat mercilessly.

Can't you remember? You went to the toilets. You hid in one. Its door ajar. Remember now? Someone came in. Another girl. You banged the door on her head. Knocked her unconscious. Then you hit her again and again with a metal rod. Till her head was chillingly unrecognisable. Spurted blood, alarmingly patterned the toilet walls. Then, a dark red puddle wrapped the floor. And you ran. You ran like crazy and dived into the nearest pool. You left all traces of her DNA in there. For an instant, you didn't mind being wet. Remember? No? Strange, because we do.

And the voices repeat themselves again and again. Each time, they get louder. Like they always do. They start as no more than a whisper and they gradually grow in strength, till they are thunderous.

I'm petrified and hyperventilating. Panic kicks in with no remorse and I find myself spinning and spinning, without control. Though this time I seem to be flying off a merry-go-round and I take a dive onto the floor until I can get my bearings. For the walls are mobile, rotating faster than I can even breathe. And I grab the leg of the bed like all hope is lost for me. I hold on tightly as can be because I sink. I submerge further and further into the seas of torment that flow turbulently through my mind. And I run without notion and vomit the bile that refuses to stay in my oesophagus, this time. I throw it all out, alarming those who can hear me retch.

Then, still, without notion, I come face to face with my mother, who is running towards me, her face disturbingly anxious.

"Mum," I wail desperately. "I've murdered someone - a girl, I think."

Chapter 20

Sandy

A fearful Mazy approaches me. All colour drained from her face. Her look is one of desperation, mixed with sheer horror. And it scares me so. She's about to collapse physically and mentally more so. I barely hear her through her wails of distress but I know what she is saying and I grab hold of her before she plunges to the floor.

"Mazy," I almost stammer. My voice is trembling. My hands too. I hear myself say, "You need professional help now. We've waited long enough, thinking that you would overcome those thoughts in your mind. Your habits. Those rituals we observe you do. But we were only fooling ourselves. We can't wait any longer. You are getting worse by the day." And I break down too, weeping bitterly, whilst I hug her tightly. Caressing her as I should have done more often, but never did.

And Mazy opens up like she has never done before. She pours out her suffering, her intolerable pain. The mumbled chain of words that tumble out of her mouth spit, all at once, the venom that stops her from leading a life, like the teenage girl she is.

She talks about the voices, the demons as she calls them. How they enchain her will. How they forbid her to enjoy herself since she was a child. How they jeer and bully her senses, until she succumbs to them, in both body and mind.

"And they always win, no matter what," she continues hysterically. "They know how to get their revenge. They started with my toys, my room, and the door that has to be locked at all times. The key. I need to check. Again and again. The rain and the dampness will ruin my bedroom and my belongings. Robbers will come and rip me off everything. The lights, the locks, the oven, the hob - all need to be switched off. A fire can break out and my room will go up in flames. My hands - they have to be impeccably clean or the germs will come in thousands.

So I check and continue to check. Till they are satisfied. But they never are. And now the worst is to come. I don't know how but I ignored them for once, just once. I listened to music and ignored their voices. Just that once, I disobeyed them. I did not listen. I felt so liberated for such a short while. But now they hit back. They take revenge. And everything escalates. They tell me now I've killed someone. A girl. They say it's a girl. But I don't remember. My mind is so fuzzy, I cannot think straight. The police, my God! They'll be after me now. I want to kill myself. End this misery and I don't know how…" Mazy's voice trails off, as she sobs inconsolably.

"My poor, poor Mazy," I almost howl, through tears of anguish. Through the years I could see the storm drawing closer by the day. But when it does, it always catches you unawares, hitting you straight in the face, with full-blown force. Because there's always more beneath the surface than you imagine. And I continue to gently caress Mazy's hair, feeling her locks escape through my fingers, just as her life seems to be escaping from her.

"The pain you are enduring so silently, for so long, will definitely go and you will lead the life you deserve," I fervently tell her, secretly not knowing if I actually believe that.

"You'll see - because this stops here and now. I'll seek immediately, the professional help I should have sought when you first started to get worse. I shouldn't have ignored it. I should have acted sooner and you wouldn't have had to face this torture on your own."

The guilt overpowers my will but it does not paralyse it any more. For now, I have extreme clarity on how I will proceed. Nothing, absolutely nothing will stop me from booking Mazy, the first appointment with the best psychiatrist, I can find.

"You haven't killed anyone Mazy. If you are not sure of anything - *be sure of that.*" I stress these words over and over, with great conviction because *that* I do believe.

"No one can get away with committing a murder in a public place, overcrowded and in broad daylight. Mazy, it's your mind escalating more and more. Confusing you to your limits. You may be hounded by demons but you've got us too, right behind you, Mazy, to keep you from falling, till you are able to stand firm and on your own. You are also surrounded by family, friends. Even angels and loved ones passed away, your spiritual guardians, and they, too, will help you through this rough and tedious journey. Don't you think for a moment that you are on your own. Don't forget it. My poor, poor, beautiful Mazy…" My voice is silent as the words are knotted in my throat. I can no longer speak, with such inexplicable sadness, that is so shockingly oppressive.

Her eyes meet mine slowly and I can see, in her gaze, a mixture of relief. Yet a fear so palpable, with somewhat disbelief, or scepticism of everything I am saying.

She wants to tell me so, I know, but I hush her gently, whilst I rock her in my arms, assuring her with all my strength, in the hope that she will change the chip for so long encrusted in her mind and somehow be 'reborn' again.

Chapter 21

Ella

Congratulations, love! You've finally achieved it. You've brought yourself to the point of collapse. You've now got the family where you want to have them, in the palm of your hand. You drama queen! I bet you're gloating that everyone is fussing over you.

You're driving Mum and Dad out of their wits, while you secretly chuckle to yourself over the whole situation, I bet. To say nothing of Freya. She's so worried about you, she's fretting like you are about to commit suicide.

My goodness, *you*! Just look at you. Everyone is at your beck and call. Has anyone asked me how I feel about all this secretive matter? Ever since it started? NO! And why would they anyway, when I know they don't care?

Ridiculous! Absolutely ridiculous! The situation is getting so out of hand. Finally, she's got Mum phoning a shrink. Let's see where that takes her. Or more likely, what further problems will that create? She's out to break up the family and slowly but surely, she's pulling it off.

There's nothing wrong with her at all. She's attention-seeking, like always. Ever since we were kids, she's had Mum revolving round her. Making me look as if I'm the black sheep of the family. Ba! Ba! Black sheep, that's who I am and I don't want to change at all to be like her. No way! I'd rather be cold, cruel and unsympathetic. I don't care because I know what I am, *real. Totally realistic.*

Mazy magnifies everything. That's exactly what she does. I keep saying it. But no one listens. Not even Freya, not anymore. She's completely taken in by Mazy. Giving her support and so much reassurance, it's pathetic. I'm going to have to feign some mental disorder or ill health myself, if anything, just to get a third of the attention Mazy enjoys. Otherwise, I know I pass absolutely unnoticed in this family.

"That's not true, Ella," Freya retorts firmly, when I get a chance to bring up the subject. I'm automatically shut up. They won't even hear me out. She says she doesn't recognise me. She doesn't like the Ella I'm turning into. Can't understand why I am so ruthless with my own flesh and blood, yet so sympathetic to other people's problems. For someone who's always been on my side, I'm the one who can't understand Freya's attitude now.

In the end, I guess she only wants me by her side when she needs me. Like when at school. She certainly needs me then, so that I can defend her, when necessary.

"Keep the bullies at bay, Ella," she'll plead. And that's when Ella comes in to save the day. Isn't that what all this is about, Freya? Yet when I need some support in this family, neither Freya nor Mum and often, not even Dad will hear me out. Especially if it's to do with dear old Mazy.

Well! All this just sucks. Life sucks. I'm so fed up, I really can't take anymore. Just longing to get my ass out of here. Can't wait. I'll go off one day and never look back. That much I do know.

Part Two

Chapter 22

Mazy

I sit in a dreary, light, green-walled room. Everything around is tired looking. The flaking paint, the aged desk, the unstable chairs that make you sit up rigidly, blatantly surfacing my uneasiness. Even the drab curtains on the windows behind the grotesque desk have seen happier times.

I guess that's why the walls are covered with posters, I can't be bothered to read. They hide all evidence of wear and tear. I cringe at the thought that this could happen to my bedroom walls. So, I look away and see my mother, tense and apprehensive, next to me. And I don't think it's the chair that is doing that.

I don't want to do the same as those posters and hide what I am feeling. Now I've started, I cannot be stopped. I've got to cascade my innermost feelings, my fears and my thoughts, to someone who can give me some steering. I thought I could navigate alone through the tempest. But not anymore, not without help. I'm aware of that much. I've never dared disclose my secrets, but now I realise there's no other way to go.

The psychiatrist walks in hurriedly. He mumbles some kind of apology for the wait, the interminable wait and my mother forces a smile, despite her uneasiness. I study him like I study everyone. Is this the person I'm about to reveal my secrets to?

Those secrets I have kept solely to myself since I was two. I'm not so sure now.

I see a pair of beady eyes, somewhat hooded, behind some worn-out specs. He can't be doing overly well, otherwise, he'd spruce up the place and also himself, I end up wondering. I'm not so sure this is a good idea, anymore.

They seem kind though, those beady, hooded eyes. I steal another look. I see his shoulder-length, dishevelled, salt-and-pepper hair, framing a noticeably angled jaw line. And this time, he's looking at me, ready to begin the session. His voice sounds calm and reassuring. I like that instantly. It gives me the surge of confidence I so need right now. Maybe this man can actually help, I tell myself. I have to grant him the benefit of the doubt, at least. Little do I know that he will become my confidant in the years to follow.

Robert James Barton. The psychiatrist introduces himself, though there's no need. He invites me to begin. My mother eyes me warily, still uneasy. She sits quietly, allowing me to relay my problems. Only stepping in from time to time, to help me find that adequate word or phrase, that makes me hesitate or stammer. I stop now and then, not only for a breather but to see the psychiatrist's reaction. Any facial expression that might dishearten me to continue. But there's none. Only eyes completely focused on me, urging me to carry on. And I do just that. I continue relating every detail of what is so deeply buried in my mind, in my heart, in my soul, wherever. What keeps me awake, more nights than I dare remember.

I finish after what seems like a lifetime. I realise I am sweating. My fringe sticks to my forehead. The chronological account of everything I've gone through leaves me absolutely exhausted. Though funnily enough, I feel good, inexplicably good. Must be the weight on my shoulders has finally lifted. I am liberated.

It's his turn to speak. I wait impatiently while he makes his notes. I notice he hasn't until now. He turns his head away from the monitor to me.

"Obsessive, compulsive disorder, OCD," he sums everything up in three words. The years of torment, the torture, the misery, the demons in my mind, all summarised in three words. Surely, no one can believe that!

"A severe case of OCD, known as Pure O," he continues. "That explains your invasive thoughts." He goes on to give examples of the common and not-so-common symptoms. Yet nothing surprises me, for I know I've lived through each and every experience he mentions. He asks me questions. He's more interested in my suicidal thoughts than anything else. He has to be sure that I won't attempt anything crazy, I guess. I reassure him.

"Suicide has been on my mind, true, but I can't bring myself to do it. I'm too much of a coward," I confess. He reckons I'm the opposite. I'm strong, he says. I'm facing my problems, not running away from them. I want to believe him, but I don't know how I'll feel tomorrow, or the day after. He explains further, though briefly, how the brain works. Brain chemistry, he calls it. He talks about my having an imbalance of serotonin, a chemical that affects emotional states.

Mum sits there numbed, her face a picture of despair and gloom. Or is it guilt that is bombarding her? She realises, no doubt, how oblivious she is and has been, to the magnitude of the mental pain I endure. I want to turn around to her and hug her. Tell her it's not her fault. But I, too, am numb to emotions. It's so hard for me to open up and I've already opened up enough these past two days. Everything has suddenly taken such a turn, it's very difficult for me to assimilate.

I'm secretly relieved that there's a name to my condition. All I want to know is that with appropriate medication, administered wisely and accurately, I can certainly lead a perfectly normal life. I want to expel those demons that blur my will, out of my life for good.

This psychiatrist, Robert James Barton, with more of an actor's name than anything, should better get it right because, for once in my lifetime, I finally see a ray of light at the end of the tunnel. I know it won't be easy, but nothing can be worse than the hardship I've lived up to now, alone and in such fear.

Chapter 23

Sandy

Why is it I feel like a train has run me over? I'm shattered and totally exhausted as if I can take no more. I should be feeling hopeful now that at least action has finally been taken. Instead, I feel so very, very miserable. Like it's been the saddest day I can remember in a long time.

I know I should be feeling positive now. Dr Barton made it all seem very clear and straight forward. He is confident that the right dosage of Setrolin will balance her serotonin levels and Mazy can, at last, start to lift off. Live her life. Enjoy herself and have fun. Have a different mindset. Yet I feel so down. A heartache that seems even physical. Like a life losing battle to a much-dreaded illness. And, as always, I cannot allow Mazy to perceive these feelings of anguish, that suddenly engulf me.

Eric embraces me tenderly. "It's hearing Mazy pour her heart out to the psychiatrist. Learning about her suicidal thoughts. Everything we've so terribly dreaded, becoming so alarmingly real. Mazy could have committed suicide and we were inexplicably oblivious to that reality. It makes you feel so shamefully guilty and impotent, I know. That's why you are feeling the way you are," he rightfully concludes.

Eric knows me well. I know he is absolutely right. Being aware of the mental problem that Mazy has carried since her early years and, seeing it worsen day by day, makes it no easier, when you hear it in first person, directly from the sufferer. Each word, each moment, so vividly described, every bit of frightful pain lived and relived. The magnitude of the problem is suddenly revealed. Laid out in front of you, like I saw it gradually developing, all these years, and it suddenly hits you, right in the face. Everything so dreaded is a bitter reality, stinging and excruciating like a spear, penetrating your heart and beyond your heart, your soul.

And all I want to do is shout. I want to shout so loud. With luck, I shall explode and disintegrate. It's the impotence that smothers and chokes me. I don't know what's harder, being the sufferer or the sufferer's mother.

When, why, and how is all I keep asking myself again and again. Was she born like this? Is it something I did or eat or didn't do or didn't eat when I was pregnant? Did I give her the right nutrients when she was growing inside of me? Did it happen during childbirth? Did I push the right way or did I push when I was told not to? Did I damage something in her brain as a result? Her brain chemistry? Aren't most mental disorders developed as a result of a lack of chemicals in the brain? That's how the psychiatrist explained it. Is it hereditary? His family or mine? In both families, there are traits of depression, anxiety, and mood swings. So, could she have inherited all this?

The exhaustion in my mind wears me down, more than all the physical commotion of the day. The web of emotions is overwhelming to the point that I must switch off, lest I collapse. I know, deep down, I mustn't seek a logical explanation for Mazy's mental disorder. It won't alleviate anything or anyone. This is something I have to live with and endure. For Mazy's sake, I must be strong. Remain positive. Be there when she needs words of comfort and encouragement. And most importantly, shower her with love. Lots of it, I know.

My mind falls on Freya and Ella. It won't be easy for them either. They too must understand what all this entails. Loads of patience and understanding on the part of everyone. We are all in this together. No selfishness, please.

And more and more thoughts continue to drift in and out of my mind. Is this what Mazy experiences every minute of the day? It's a wonder she isn't crazy yet. I would be. I'll go crazy if this long day, which has paved its way to the longest night ever, doesn't end soon.

The dawn comes out of nowhere and I haven't yet slept a wink. I drag myself out of the bed. Heavier in heart than ever.

Chapter 24

Freya

I flutter around everyone nowadays. I'm here and there for all. Possibly like always. Though now it seems as if it's round the clock. No time to think about me, really. This is not about how I feel. Not now anyway. I must give my support to everyone. They are all so lost, suddenly.

Mum, I know she's getting a piece of the aftermath. I need to be there for her. She feels so guilty. I tell her not to be and she smiles slowly at me, with eyes that say something else. She caresses my hair and touches my face gently, with genuine gratitude and although she continues with a positive attitude, I know she believes differently.

Dad, poor, poor Dad! It's hard to tell just how bad he feels. He's good at hiding problems. Work-related ones, in particular. I know he's suffering terribly in silence. Doesn't want to upset Mum more than she already is. I hear them speaking softly at night, in the privacy of their bedroom. They think we are all sleeping but I'm not. I hear them. Reassuring words of comfort is what I hear but, I know they are hurting badly. They argue too, often. Who can blame them? The situation is not easy to bear, day in and day out. It tires even the tireless, at some given point.

Ella? Amazing how she won't budge an inch from her way of thinking. Not even now that Mazy has a diagnosis for the mental stress she has dragged along, and even dragged *us* along, for as far as can be remembered. She's strong-willed our Ella is. I'm sure she'd feel some sympathy for a friend, or even someone she hardly knew, who had the same problem. She's a people's friend. Someone they can trust when in trouble. Good old Ella will surely come to the rescue. Certainly not a family friend, though. That's what it looks like to me. She just won't come to understand Mazy's condition. Doesn't even try. Says she just can't tolerate Mazy's quest for drama. The eternal drama queen, she calls her. Deep down, I know Ella will come around, one day. She'll open her eyes to Mazy's reality and, possibly, become her strongest supporter. When she's older and more mature, no doubt. Though age is no excuse. Just look at me.

So, I flutter and flutter like a delicate butterfly or maybe like a hovering dragonfly, throwing light to whoever needs it the most. Mazy is surprisingly receptive to my 'light' and even welcomes it.

We sit and talk about the session with Dr Barton and she is unbelievably open about it all. I see her hopeful for the very first time, in this tedious plight. I hide the pain I feel, as I hear Mazy pour her heart out. There are so many things I was totally unaware of. I can understand now, how Mum and Dad feel. It's such a feeling of emptiness. So incredibly stomach-gripping. Similar to the grief death leaves behind. Mostly, I think it's the impotence we feel. Like a feeling of failure. We weren't able to reach out to Mazy, yet knowing there was something so very wrong with her. Words of comfort are now so necessary. I know they would be for me. I tell her we're so very, very proud of her. I include Ella too. That gives Mazy the extra boost she needs.

"Mazy, it's your time to fly now, to take off and shine. You'll dazzle everyone who gets to know you, believe me. You will," I assure her, with a big smile.

And I vehemently cross two fingers from the hand I have strongly clenched behind my back. *I so want to believe it, too.*

Chapter 25

Mazy

I'm overwhelmed. Unsure of my feelings. Feelings that are bitter-sweet. A kind of success on the one hand, but on the other, I'm petrified. Scared the demons will not be stopped by a one-pill wonder. Can I believe this? Should I get excited that a cure for my predicament is at hand? No! No! No! It's too soon to count my chickens.

Setrolin versus the *demons*, versus the *voices*, versus my *mind*. Who will win? A little pill of no more than a few milligrams, can outride my mental enemies? Too soon to tell! Far too soon! I'm scared to be hopeful. I fear I'll land once again, with yet a bigger thump.

I'll start on them tomorrow. Take it from there. I'm secretly pleased, despite my uncertainties. It felt good speaking to someone who did not judge me. Who understood and was not taken aback when I talked about the worst thought that has ever haunted me. The thought that I had killed someone. This Dr Barton made me reason with myself. Something that I have never done. He made me see the logic. As if he lifted the wool from my eyes and I managed to see with clarity. I know I must remain positive but something tells me, the clarity will be marred before long.

I'm confused. Where do I go from here? This will probably mark a turning point in my life. Before Dr Barton and after. I have a feeling I shall see a lot of this psychiatrist. He's a good listener. Not a bit judgemental. I know it's his job not to be but it's so easy to be subjective, rather than objective.

It scares me too, to think what I'm doing to my family, my parents, in particular. I feel so selfish at times. Most of the time. That's what Ella says but she's not inside my head. If only she could see what goes on within the walls of my brain. Have a little peek, at least. I'm sure she'd be more understanding and tolerant.

I'm in a reflective mood, all of a sudden. I return my thoughts to my parents. I remember the lines of the song from "Fiddler on the Roof", one of my mother's favourite musicals.

"I can't remember getting older, how then did they?"

I might have tweaked those lines slightly, I think, but they describe perfectly what I'm feeling now.

I slowly observe my Dad. I realise I have never stopped to do that. So, I haven't noticed that suddenly, he doesn't look as fit and strong as he once did. He isn't as young any more. When did that happen? He's such a hard worker. He even always works weekends to make ends meet. Never a word of protest. Forever willing and able. He made us feel so safe when we were little. His hands, large and powerful, were always there to catch us when we fell. To caress us gently and hug us. Now dry calluses are incrusted in the skin of those hands, from so much labour. Is it worthwhile, I wonder? I gaze at his silver hair, once so very black.

How much I've failed to see in all these years, that I've succumbed to the demons, and given them priority over everything else. The wrinkles too, folding and falling over sad eyes, hooding them and making them lose their spark, are somehow so visible now. Dad seemed so tall once, towering above us, but not now. Not anymore. The extra kilos gained too, without awareness or measure and the unrelenting pain of screaming joints, proclaim audaciously the scurrying age that just cannot be denied. How did I fail to see all that?

Mum too, is a tireless workaholic, both in and out of home. The recollection of her flawless complexion, clear and pale against her thick, unruly, curly hair that fell grandly over her shoulders, so similar to Grandma Aida's, rests vividly in my mind. Now, today, I see her flawless skin has welcomed various wrinkles, to sit peacefully in the crevices made by her smile. Her big eyes, tinged with cinnamon and blended with honey, generously clad with lashes, were always so very expressive. Hence the lines that have compellingly settled there as well, determined to stay, no matter the miracle cures applied. Her hair, still thick, is now highlighted and straightened, any silver trace shunned. Mum finally took control of those unmanageable curls from my childhood memories. Those rebellious curls that flew out of hand, despite a firm brush, a firm hairband or firm clips to tame them. Had she had those marvellous straighteners then!

I recall Mum's medium build, strictly disciplined not to become a large build. Mum is so very disciplined in everything really. She wakes up at six thirty sharp each day, nearly always beating the alarm. Never lingering in bed not even on a cold, dismal winter's morn; and then she just gets on with it. That's Sandy, my Mum, she just makes things happen.

It's a long time since I took a breather and eyed carefully those around me. Those who truly love me. *Those* who are truly important. When I have a moment of 'peace' within, like now, though that isn't very often, I realise the hurt, the sheer pain I'm causing all of them. I want to change but I just can't. I cannot put a stop to this misery. All I can say is that I sincerely hope this wonder drug can conquer the demons and chuck them out for good. Keep them dormant at least, though I know they don't even nap.

Chapter 26

Sandy

I feel slightly better. Still going through a haphazard chain of emotions but gradually feeling more positive. The visit to the psychiatrist was a really good move if ever there was one. I feel half the battle is now won. Still a long, winding road ahead, though. Undoubtedly, full of obstacles around each bend. It won't be any easier than the previous stretch lived, I know. But this time, I feel ready and more prepared for the 'enemy'. The volcano won't erupt on me this time.

It was terrifying to see how Mazy was progressively getting worse. Lately, in massive leaps and bounds. I couldn't postpone it any more. I *had* to take action. Otherwise, the inevitable would have happened. Now I have faith that this medication will steadily begin to play its part. It'll help to lift her depression as well, or so Dr Barton assures. He was scared to administer anything else that may give Mazy more suicidal thoughts, considering to my utmost dismay, she confessed to having them.

I'm sure Mazy is expecting Setrolin to be the miracle cure we are all hoping for, and it probably is, but over considerable time, I guess. I'll tell her to be patient. Miracles don't happen overnight but they *do* happen. And I want her to believe in them. Like any mother, I can't wait to see my daughter blooming in health, in every shape or form. To finally take control and start life's journey. I want to see her enjoy herself with family and friends. Carefree, untroubled, serene. Be the family we all want to be. Not half a family. I'm glad we are still together, though. So many families in similar situations, just fall apart. Go their separate ways. They can't take the uncertainties, the hardship that is endured, practically the twenty four hours of each day.

I can't imagine my life without Eric's support in this. It's such a blessing he's there when needed. Mazy is not the only one who requires reassurance. We all do at some precise moment. Though he's a man of few words, he's aware of what's going on around him. Actions for him speak louder than words. He's been my rock and I need him to stay that way. I feel so sorry for those people who face all kinds of adversities alone, totally on their own. How they can get up and confront each day, knowing that there's no one at home to offer comfort and encouragement, I'll never know. I take my hat off to these people. People who start with a strong relationship, a beautiful home and a marvellous family, and gradually they see how their whole world tumbles, like a tower built from a pack of cards.

I've learned to appreciate a kind word or gesture so very, very much. However minimal, it doesn't matter, it's still so incredibly great. Taking it for granted is such a big mistake. I used to do that, practically all the time but not anymore. Amazing how we change. Mature? Possibly. We never stop learning. Life is such a learning journey. And we don't have to be in any school to learn the hardest and most important lessons. The classes are just out there, as we climb out of bed each morning and live through the day as it unfolds.

Chapter 27

Mazy

The months that follow bring with them a blizzard of sensations, that are totally new for me. Everyone eyes me cautiously, wondering whether or not the Setrolin is kicking in. I eye them back defiantly, wanting to shout at the top of my voice, "***STOP IT!*** I can't be studied like a lab mouse!" Don't they understand that nothing will cure my mind? Don't they realise that I could be partying, clubbing, dancing, singing, yet my mind is miles away, immersed in the most remote, black pit, where the surface is always beyond reach?

My life continues to dangle dangerously from a thread, confused with my new situation, yet secretly excited and expectant. I must admit that I feel less depressive now. I even develop a dry sense of humour I never knew I had. I feel more confident. Confident to do things. I don't even know if this sudden motivation is real or surreal. I know one thing, I'm scared to be happy. Scared to feel positive, because I don't know if the high I'm experiencing, will be subsequently replaced by the abhorrent feeling of doom, I so much dread.

Girl meets music once again. And this time it becomes her ally.

Yep! That's something I can *fervently* vow. Music saves me from my worst enemy, that *MIND* of mine. It doesn't conquer it, though. The enemy is still there, ready to pounce on me at any given moment. But I want music in my life and there's no stopping me. No more bizarre voices ringing in my ears, telling me I cannot play music or sing and dance to the beat, only the voices of the singers I choose to hear. There can't be limitations, not with music. Not like last time. Bring back NIRVANA, I say. Listening to them is my religion. I cannot understand though, why I can't be as strong, as to deafen every demon's voice, permanently.

I take up music at school and I realise I *can* sing. I can actually stand up in front of a class and sing. ME! I couldn't do that a few months back. It boosts my confidence so very much, I'm in high spirits. *Me, yes, me*! It seems impossible for me to feel a ray of hope and happiness, but the truth is I feel it. Erratically, but I feel it.

Not much later come the concerts, the band I form, the song-writing; those beautiful lyrics that flow, almost magically, as I strum the strings of my mother's old guitar. That guitar, propped up in a corner of her bedroom for as long as I can remember. The same one that has stared at me from its leather case all these years, until I took the plunge. I teach myself to play. It's easy now that I realise I have an ear for music.

I spend my days in our band room, rehearsing amidst technically advanced sound systems, sophisticated microphones and diverse musical instruments. It becomes my other 'sanctuary.' I know this one has to be shared, so I struggle to relax.

It's not my bedroom, I keep telling myself. It's hard to do. The more I go, the more at ease I feel in there, and the harder it becomes.

OK Stop it now. I warn myself.

No one will steal these instruments. No one has the key to the place. The place is not yours. Not everything in there, belongs to you.

And before I have a chance to check myself, my monsters race ahead of me.

It's an old place. Is there water ingress? Will it rain tomorrow? Will the rain seep through and ruin the stuff inside? Are the cables safe? No short circuit to spark off a fire?

Check! CHECK! ***CHECK!***

What about that wonder drug? What the hell is it doing? I bet my demons are chuckling their heads off now.

Chapter 28

Sandy

I ask Eric if he sees a change in Mazy. He says he does. So do I. She speaks to us, that's the difference. Before, she was totally withdrawn. Only spoke when she had to. No life in those words. No spark. No oomph. There's no nothingness now when I observe her gaze. Even when she's lost in thought, I still see something that wasn't there before. Not for as long as I can remember. Now I see hope. I cross my fingers. I want to continue seeing hope coming out of those eyes. I want to see them expressive and meaningful. That can only mean that Mazy is motivated. That she has an incentive to move forward. That the demoralised state she's usually in will vanish, if not immediately, through time. I pray that she's consistent from now on. I don't want her to give up. Not ever.

She seems happier in school, too. No longer that zombie, forced to get out of bed each morning. I know Freya sees it as well. I don't want to share my feelings with Mazy too much, in case she thinks we are constantly observing her. I'm sure she already thinks it. So, I measure my words and also my steps, for fear Mazy misinterprets them and comes to the wrong conclusions. The last thing I want to do now is affect her progress. Halt it in any way. It's hard though. It's as if I can't be myself. Unable to say or do what I really want to say and do. I'm usually so spontaneous over everything and everyone. Now I feel my words and actions are studied and rehearsed and I hate that.

Eric reckons it won't be for long and as always, his words are encouraging. As long as Mazy has an incentive, she's on the right path, he assures. He's right as always. Seeing Mazy interested in music is a fantastic way forward. She tells me so too, and I love to hear her natter away about her song-writing abilities, my old guitar or the school concerts ahead. Anything she tells me is a God-sent gift. Should I say it's *music* to my ears? Never best said!

It's great to see her get out and about more, even if it's just to the band room and back. At least she's interacting with others over a mutual interest and that's so rewarding. I really want to think that only positive thoughts currently travel in and out of Mazy's mind, so very complex until now. I *do* want that mind to break away completely from the shadows that have, so far, darkened all its corners. I *do* want it to welcome the light that is now slowly being cast.

We all have to be patient, I know. I keep telling myself that. I realise time is of the essence here and we all want to see an immediate change in Mazy's state of mind, but we'll learn to walk together before we can run. And when we can, nobody will stop us. We'll all be winners in this never-ending race.

Chapter 29

Eric

There's so much suddenly to assimilate, it's hard to take it all in. Everything seems beyond realisation. I even wonder if Sandy and I also need psychological help, despite how terribly against 'shrinks' I've always been. Notwithstanding my apprehension, I can't help but admit, that there was no other way forward. Now I can say with total conviction that Mazy's mind was fogged since the beginning of her days. Unfortunately, we could all see it getting more and more misty. I had hoped the mist would lift one day but instead, it densely obscured her will to a greater extent. It reduced her capacity to think with clarity, lately confusing her senses and cunningly planting seeds of ambiguity, where lucidity should grow.

I don't want to think that I have impeded Mazy's mental well-being by refusing any psychological treatment whatsoever. I feel so horribly vulnerable. I don't want to feel this guilt. It'll make me even more vulnerable and I must remain strong for everyone's sake. We can't all be emotional wrecks. I've said before, I don't want to be the one who takes the ship down. I need to help Sandy steer it against adversity.

"We are in this together," she reiterates tirelessly. "And together we must see it through."

So, I stand tall, in case I fall. I must be like Freya. She gives us constant moral support. I'm so proud of her. I want to think that Ella too, can understand this situation and show some sympathy. I'm sure she will. I'll speak to her about it. She'll understand, no doubt.

There must be so many families similarly afflicted and possibly living through more precarious situations than us, bearing the brunt of it all in silence, enduring the hardship alongside the sufferer. I expect someday, we'll get in touch with those likewise affected and share our experiences, offering each other mutual support. For now, I feel I cannot share these personal circumstances. I know Sandy feels the same way. I'm sure many must disagree with our decision, but I'm scared of how the consequences will affect Mazy. How it will affect all of us. It's early days and we are all a little lost. Unsure and scared of the outcome.

At this precise moment, we must be wary. Watch our steps as we tread on eggshells. Any false move and Mazy can dangerously regress instead of progress. We must continue to be patient. Where this patience comes from, beats me. I shall never know, because just when I think I've lost practically all the tolerance that can possibly exist inside a person, my persistence grows unbelievably stronger. It must be that I realise I am not alone. Otherwise, I would crumble and my life would crush, without the slightest hope of rebirth. I must keep going for everyone's sake and I pray fervently each day, that Mazy keeps going too.

Battle those enemies inside your head, Mazy. Don't let them get the better of you. Fight them with whatever strength is left in you. If our patience grows steadily on, so must your strength. Show them who's in command. YOU, NOT THEM!

Chapter 30

Ella

Why is everyone expecting me to be empathetic? I don't want to be. I don't understand Mazy and I don't want to either. It's such a chore, it's overwhelming.

I bet no one knows I'm unhappy at school. No, of course not. Why would they? Their whole world revolves around Mazy. Besides, am I not the popular one? The one with no problems. The one who leads, who decides. The one whom everyone follows. Well, not anymore. Since I moved to secondary, there are many who want to lead. They hate my popularity, so they hate me because they are envious. It's become a competition, I don't want any part in it.

I don't even try to be popular. I just attract people. I don't do anything special.

Just laugh. It must be that. I laugh easily. It must be contagious because I set everybody off. I'm witty too, so I shut them up abruptly before they even have a chance to open their stupid mouths. That's what they find annoying. Those who want to pick on me, give up, because I chuckle and giggle so much, it defeats their purpose. And their anger spirals uncontrollably. I know they can't stand me.

To add to all this, I must look out for Freya. I can't let these bitches take it out on her, just because they can't get to me. I tell Freya to keep an eye out for them. She knows who they are and what they get up to. I know she worries about me too. Tells me to keep away from them.

Can't wait to leave school, honestly. Not because of the bitches, really. But because this is not for me. I've come to realise I'm not academic. I hate studying. I have no study skills, whatsoever. No favourite assignment. Don't even have a clue about what I'd like to do in the future. No idea. No motivation either. I'll keep this from Mum for now. The last thing I want to do is burden her with unnecessary problems. I know Mum will go livid when she finds out I want to quit school. She's aware of my difficulty to study, but she's got lots of hope I'll transition into the perfect student, as I get older. I'll let her worry about Mazy for now. She's got enough on her plate with her. The rest is on me. I know I can keep my 'enemies' under control.

And when I get home, I'll keep out of everyone's way, too. I'll avoid confrontations with Mazy. But I can't promise anything, because if she rubs me up the wrong way, I know I'll explode. I won't wait patiently for almost three hours, till she finishes in the bathroom. No way. She'd better be the last one in, otherwise, I cannot guarantee a storm won't break out.

I can't even bring myself to ask Mazy about her appointment with the psychiatrist. I think that's who she visited. I don't even feel guilty about that. Everyone urges me to do so but I just can't. How can she listen to her mind the way she does? It just doesn't make sense. She's going to ruin her life if she continues this way. I hear she's on medication now. I bet she'll be on it for life. Is this what you want for yourself, Mazy? What on earth are you doing? What a way to go.

Mazy and her mind! Get your act together, girl!

Chapter 31

Mazy

Can a parrot take the monsters away from my head? Is that what they think? Do they actually think that an African Grey to be exact, can make the demons in my head vanish? Is this another wonder drug like Setrolin? Sometimes I wonder who's actually suffering from a mental disorder. Me or them? I can't understand it. Mum doesn't like us to have pets. Says it's an extra responsibility she can do without. Moneywise, too, because it's an additional expense we just can't afford. That's why everybody is so awed when Dad comes in, one evening, with a haughty madam in a colossal cage. I have to look twice because I can't believe what I am seeing.

"This is Polly," Dad beams as he announces her name, though his expression soon changes when he eyes Mum. "A friend of mine couldn't keep her anymore. Didn't have the time to look after her properly…"

"And do you think we have?" Mum snaps before he can finish his sentence. "Where on earth shall we place this cage? I don't want this big bird, and her equally gigantic cage, in everybody's way. How long is she staying?" Mum starts off nagging, to everyone's disappointment, as Polly has taken over our attention completely.

Does Mum change her mind when she sees how impacted I am by Polly? Does she think that my unexpected enthusiasm might make me forget my mental disorder? Does Dad actually bring Polly home, at such a significant time, to ease the tension we are all feeling and clear the atmosphere a little?

I admit Miss Polly has me totally devoted to her that summer. She winds me round her little claw and without prior realisation, a strong bond is suddenly created between the two of us. When everyone is down at the beach, I am at home, alone with this parrot that will only respond to me, like I am her master. They say parrots have only one owner and that is certainly me. I suddenly have a spectator full of admiration for me. So much so that it doesn't take me long to get Polly out of her cage and let her wander freely around the house. All she wants to do is perch herself on my shoulder and tickle the side of my neck and face with her feathers. I am wary at the beginning. I think she might bite my finger off, as I caress her head softly. I am wrong, because she loves it, and even tilts her head back, so I can continue stroking her gently.

This is a good summer. A different one. I'm no longer alone, at home, as in past summers. Polly gives me a sense of duty. I clean her cage and feed her. I thought I'd find it revolting but looking after this parrot is amazingly therapeutic for me. I feel so animated, I take my guitar and strum the strings, till chords and lyrics fuse into a song. I sing to Polly, for she's my audience, filling completely my auditorium.

But wait. No! No! My bedroom door is slightly ajar. I become more careless when I'm alone because I relax. I know now I shouldn't. She catches me off guard and waddling curiously, dances into my haven. One claw, two claws. *She's in.*

NO! NO! Get out, Polly! You'll poo on my bed! There'll be germs everywhere. Get out! NOW!

I try and grab her but she flutters away. She's on my laptop table. OOOOOHHHHHHH! Now on my shelf, knocking down books and all. I jump to get hold of her, but her feathers slip through my fingers and she flaps her wings onto the top of my wardrobe. I despair.

Damn! Damn! She's playing up now. Reminds me of Ella. I think suddenly, this parrot is not such a good idea after all.

Chapter 32

Sandy

There's no pleasing Mazy. She's so fastidious, even at the best of times. Well! Looks like our dear old parrot won't be accompanying us for much longer. It's a blessing for me, really. Once summer is over, no one wants to look after Polly. They are all back at school and the poor bird is gradually neglected when routines commence. No matter how many rotas I create to clean and feed Polly, none are adhered to. Totally unfair to her, toddling in her cage, amidst tons of dried seeds and muck. What a mess and what a feast for mosquitoes! Not the ideal scenario for a busy lifestyle and certainly not for Polly.

So, unfortunately, perhaps more so for Mazy who is attached to this parrot, in her own strange way, we say goodbye to Polly, just like we said hello months back. I would hold onto this bird, even if it means my looking after her twenty-four-seven, but I realise now, Mazy's not that keen on her anymore. She's beginning to have second thoughts about Polly. I know Mazy got distressed, one day when the parrot waltzed into her room. I don't know what upset Mazy more, the fact that Polly was going to ruin her sanctuary or the fact that she was negligent enough to leave the door open.

I bet her mind did an instant reel of a full three hundred and sixty degrees. It probably blackened her senses and made her desperately hyperventilate, for her sanctuary means the world to her. Seeing the bird knock everything down, seeing her droppings land on her bed, or anywhere within those sacred bedroom walls, must be like a tough whack below the belt. Pity really, because in actual fact, I *did* think she was enjoying looking after Polly. It surprised me to see Mazy cleaning out her cage and getting her hands grubby. I was secretly pleased. Polly is helping Mazy overcome some of her obsessive compulsions, I instantly think. But my hopes are soon shattered, when she tells me, she frantically tried to shoo the parrot out of her room. I guess, *again,* we progress and regress simultaneously, and my heart sinks.

Though, sigh as I may, this is not just about the parrot, or any other pet that we could keep, for that matter. It's not even about the girls not adhering to a rota, for the poor bird's well-being. It's about Mazy changing her set ways. It's about acceptance. Learning to live together in harmony. Giving and taking in equal shares. Both family and even pets accepting each other without question or measure. But then, of course, this only happens in an ideal world. Not the world we live in. Our world. Those walls of our house. Will we ever manage to call it home? Home, Sweet Home!

In all honesty, nothing has actually changed. Mazy, may be trying, who knows, to overcome her obsessive compulsions, but she's still 'en route'. I don't want to be impatient either. There are so many obstacles we've managed to beat along the way. So now that we've all managed to catch the bull by its horns, we just cannot give up. *No way,* I say! *No way*!

Chapter 33

Mazy

I remember well those crucial, challenging years of exams. My greatest struggle, perhaps. Pushing the ogres out of my senses to let in equations, logarithms, Shakespeare, and Dickens to mention but a few, is a nightmare of its own. The invaders won't allow it. They feel superior, for they dwell permanently in every nook and cranny of my mind. Likewise, they manifest themselves.

There's no room here for anyone or anything.

I can hear their voices echoing forcefully. They can bellow louder but each blusterous word resonates a clear message that cannot be denied. My panic mode is switched on. I try frantically to snap out of my fears.

Remember the music, I desperately tell myself, as if there's another 'me' inside of me. I clutch at the smallest of straws. Call it hope, if you wish.

No worries! No worries! I reassure myself frenetically. *I won't listen to them. Like when I'm listening to music. I no longer pay attention to them, when I listen to music. I'll do so now, in the same way.*

I try so hard, it's unbelievable. I know I'll go insane at some point. Each day, each night, as I bring out my books, I'm a wrestler in a battle of wits till, completely exhausted, I can no longer arbitrate. I park everything. I put on my headphones and turn to Kurt Corbain, a hero, then, for me. For he, too, was a lost soul. His music though, is a magical balm that helps me through my darkest hours, hand in hand with Setrolin, my other 'help', supposedly.

My music class gives me a break. I look forward to concerts that loom ahead. I'll sing my heart out and feel liberated. The feeling will be so good, it will help me balance the tedious burden of studies.

My nails sting sharply as I strum the strings of the guitar. I must let them grow. I must stop inflicting pain on myself like this. My parched hands are proof enough of the pain I endure. It makes it so very difficult for me to enjoy playing.

Macbeth! Macbeth! I must return to Shakespeare. Review and summarise Dickens's Great Expectations.

"*Out, damned spot; out I say!*" shrieks Lady Macbeth in sheer desperation, whilst I apply these famous words to my invaders.

Out of my mind! Out I say, NOW! But I don't stand up strong enough. I must rebel. I did so once. I almost died when they took revenge. I must do it again; pluck up the courage to defy the wretched demons that haunt me of all power and purpose.

I move on to Dickens. Great Expectations is next. I cannot do it. I cannot concentrate. They keep on torturing me.

Go away! I want no part in your conspiracy, in your wicked plot to make me lose my wits. Let me go back to Pip and Estella, Miss Havisham and Biddy. I must rely on my photographic memory to memorise extracts from these passages, for I need to pass tomorrow's literature exam and those that follow.

I hate you, damn you! Stop telling me the walls are damp. Don't distract me from my work. NO! Rain won't seep through. My belongings will not be ruined.

I have to learn these passages by heart:

"Nobody is born a warrior.

You choose to be one when you refuse to stay seated.

You choose to be one when you refuse to back down.

You choose to be one when you stand up after getting knocked down.

You choose to be one because if not you, who?"

Famous lines I should apply to myself, this time. I thought I was a pacifist but I am a warrior, too. I'm in continuous battle and I'm tired, so very tired. How can I study in peace when my head is a battlefield and I'm on the front line, alone and defenceless?

Setrolin, which side are you on? Sometimes I doubt you are on mine.

Chapter 34

Freya

I hate exams! Can't wait to get mine out of the way. I give them my best shot. That's all I can do. I know I'll repeat a few, I'm sure, but I'm not worrying any longer. I feel so sorry for Mazy, though. Don't know how she can juggle so many things in that mind of hers. Even the concerts for which she is rehearsing, make me wonder how she can cope. I'm glad in a way that music is her escape valve. At least now, she has something worthwhile occupying her mind. Is the wonder drug doing its bit, I wonder?

Strange thing this OCD business. I can't bring myself to understand how she simply appears on stage and gets on with it. Where do her fears go? Her worries, her anxiety, where does she leave them? For somebody who frets so terribly and loses all notion of time, because of her endless rituals, how come she's completely on time when it comes to singing? Her guitar is totally tuned. Her lyrics are thoroughly learned. Her music folder, spick and span. Why isn't she like that for everything else? Absolutely inexplicable! Mazy never fails to amaze me.

But now, I'm more concerned about Ella than Mazy, believe it or not. She's going through a rough patch. I know she worries about me too, but I tell her not to. I think I can now look after myself, better than she can. That's what happens when you are used to popularity. When you don't have it, it's like turning from riches to rags. Who would have thought that being so popular would suddenly be detrimental? Envy! Always envy! That's what does it. It creeps stealthily up people's spines and sticks to them like gum, for the rest of their lives. If people turned green each time they felt envious or jealous, goodness, how many tinted people there'd be!

The upsetting thing about all this is that Ella has decided to quit school at the end of this year. When Mum finds out, she'll go crazy. I try to reason with her, like always. Good old Freya to the rescue; to talk some sense into her and whoever needs it. Like always, too, she won't hear anyone. She's absolutely steadfast in her decision. Jesus! Why can't people be like me? I *can* reason. Why do they complicate life for themselves and for everyone else, when life itself is already so very complicated?

"Ella, whatever are you going to do if you quit now? Who's going to employ you? You're still too young. At least do so after the exam results, if you must. What if you need to repeat as I'll probably have to?" I tirelessly insist, but all my pleading falls on deaf ears. I can't imagine anyone being so oblivious to reality.

Now where do I go from here? Can't tell Mum. Ella will have to, if and when she goes ahead with this. I could tell Dad but I don't want to upset him. He already has his fair share. Mazy, then? Will Mazy want to listen? I don't think so. As much as I hate to admit it, this disorder is making Mazy really selfish. She only thinks about herself and her problems. Besides, she's got enough on her plate with all the exams she's got in the coming weeks.

I'll have to continue pestering Ella. One way or another, I need to knock some sense into her. And *pronto*!

Chapter 35

Eric

Is that Mazy I'm seeing on stage? Yes, it is! But I can't believe it's her. It's absolutely incredible. Just a few weeks back, I can honestly say, Mazy seemed lifeless. Existing more than living. Anything we said to encourage her was a complete waste of time. She refused to hear us. Totally ignored us. I tried so hard to make her break down. Cry. Shout. Whatever. If only to get some reaction. But she never reacted. I know she was suffering. I wanted to help her badly as her mother did, but to no avail. Our efforts were fruitless. Instead, I cried silently in impotence. In frustration, too.

Now I see this young lady, standing tall and grand, on a stage that seems to welcome her perfectly. Like she was always part of it. And she's no longer that unresponsive person she was becoming. So indifferent, it made me squirm in silent anguish. I so hope she's past that. Hope she can now move forward positively, in whatever direction she chooses but with the will and determination, that just wasn't there before.

I have to admit that some good has come from her visit to the psychiatrist. The medication, too, seems to be gradually scoring points, because the change in her is quite obvious. Mazy will continue to visit this man regularly, for now. If he is her miracle worker, then, so be it. I finally have faith that he will clear her senses and bring them out of the darkness. I *hate* to see Mazy upset. Can't bear to see her wince and cringe in fear and torment, only because, unknowingly, I accidentally interrupt her rituals. Those wretched compulsions, so very demanding. We kept seeing them develop more and more. Enveloping Mazy, till they almost devoured her.

I think of her exams and I'm concerned for her again. She's coping alright, though. I ask Sandy and she reassures me Mazy seems to be managing surprisingly well. Better than ever before. It all seems surreal. Are we winning? Should I still be sceptical? Is she hiding anything from us, really? If only I could get inside her head. If only I could change her chip. Reprogram her mind with positivity and optimism. Ingrain them there for good.

The song she sings echoes through the hall. Her voice, so powerful yet so melodious, blends in harmony with the music she plays. It's like a breath of fresh air that caresses your skin. She captivates her audience, too. It's so relaxing to hear her. Is it the same voice that screams blue murder at Ella? The same voice that argues incessantly, that we can't even have a meal in peace and quiet, whilst simultaneously, being totally unresponsive to us.

Who are you, Mazy? I confess I don't really know you. You catch me by surprise each time. This today is a *pleasant* surprise. I never knew you had it in you. Tell me, what other surprises do you have in store for us? When you step down from the stage and go back to your other 'world', will I see you linger in corners? Carrying out those unnecessary rituals, I cannot bring myself to understand, no matter how I try. I'll sigh, just like Sandy sighs and think we are not there yet.

Give her time, I'll say. *All that she needs.*

Chapter 36

Mazy

My messed up world changes abruptly. I become more active than ever before. The mess continues, though. I always say there's a before and after, with regards to Dr Robert Barton. I shall never forget him, never in this lifetime and even in the next! The first psychiatrist I ever visit and I bond with him immediately, despite my initial apprehension. I visit him regularly, thereafter. It does me a world of good just being there. Even if I don't know what to say and I stammer and falter like a fool, I know he listens. Or he talks and I listen. No fuss, no tension, no judgement. I can open up completely, no matter what invasive thoughts hover in my mind, haunting my senses.

He shares my passion for music. He's from the Beatle-mania years but, no problem, because I enjoy classics, too. I tell him the demons are still there. Powerful and dominant, they strike back at me, without remorse.

"Keep busy," he declares with fervour. "Whilst you are active, you are winning the game. No problem if the voices continue, because they can't stop you now from doing whatever you want. They can't 'paralyse' you like they did before, because slowly but surely, you are getting mentally stronger. Soon you'll show them who's boss; who leads the show. And the voices will get weaker. One day you won't even hear them, even if you stop to listen. Don't forget they are not even voices that you hear, they are thoughts that invade your vulnerable mind."

He gives my confidence such a boost, like an energy drink, zooming through my veins and making my heart pound. His calming words are the get-up-and-go antidote I need. More precise than any medication. Yet he tells me to continue with Setrolin. "It will help with your depression," he adds. I nod in agreement. I know I often doubt the powers of the wonder drug but, I must admit, I *do* feel different since I've been taking this pill. I guess, Setrolin must be at work, levelling the serotonin in my brain, though my emotions are still haywire. There's so much I still don't understand.

True, I would never have the nerve to sing on stage otherwise. I didn't even know I had a good singing voice, let alone an ear for music. How long have I seen my mother's guitar in its brown leather case, gathering dust? Never would I have thought, one day, I would teach myself to play and that I would sing along to its strum, in synchronised rhythm and beat. How would I have formed a band, otherwise? Or play in the town square with thousands gathering round, dancing, singing in harmonised rhythm and pace? It's a great feeling to see so many people enjoying themselves, and I can't believe it's thanks to my music and songs.

It's so gratifying when they approach me to say I was great. I needed this, I reckon. It's time I, too, took a long, relishing bite into the apple and not just have it dangling from a string before my very mouth, unable to sink my teeth into it. Not *this* time.

It's how I meet Ethan, too. He likes the covers I do. Some from Blink 182, others from a variety of artists we both follow. We talk long and slow and enjoy each other's company. He stays behind to help the group gather our music equipment. And he stayed by my side from that day on. Until the inevitable happens.

Chapter 37

Sandy

For once I feel so optimistic. I see Mazy's progress and I'm delighted at the change I'm observing. *OK, be wary!* I know I can't count my chickens yet, but nobody can dispute this positive transformation, that just cannot go unnoticed. It's the change I was waiting for. A chance for her to spread her wings. I don't care if music is the reason, or Setrolin is the cause. Whichever it is, it's a god-damn blessing!

I was the proudest person on earth in that school hall, on the day of the concert. To say nothing of the concerts in the town square or the jamming in local clubs and pubs. I'm there. In the front row. No one will stand in my way or obscure my view, because I'll push them to one side, with every bit of strength there's left in me. That voice of hers that has been silent for so long, has finally spoken up. In song. Like it's woken up suddenly from many winters' hibernations. And I don't care if you tell me to watch out, because now I am *ecstatic*. Overjoyed. Like nothing I have ever felt in all my life. I want to enjoy the feeling. I want to believe in her and I want the rest of the family to believe in her, too.

This time I just don't care if Mazy relapses, because I know she can make the effort to pick herself up again and continue. To come out of the profound. To juggle many things at the same time, like studies, exams and concerts and still manage to keep her head above the water. Most importantly, she is showing us, with all the courage that is in her, that she has the will to succeed. The number of people she's meeting, the beginnings of new friendships, it's everything I wanted for Mazy. And I'm absolutely chuffed. No! No! I won't be scared to feel chuffed. Not this time. I've been scared for too long. So now I AM CHUFFED!

And I hear there's a special friend. An Ethan, if I'm informed correctly by Freya. Eric is a little apprehensive. He says there are too many changes happening all at once. It can be detrimental for Mazy. Can it? And the years Mazy has been alone, fighting her demons till they were undefeatable? Was that not more detrimental to her? I don't know if Ethan will be good or bad for Mazy. Maybe he has come at the right time or then, maybe not. Who knows anything, unless we have a crystal ball before us? All I know is that I want to see Mazy as I'm seeing her now. Active. Motivated. With determination to move forward. To become well.

If Ethan can help her recover, then he's more than welcome. Mazy's no fool. She'll soon realise if this lad is good for her or not. For a first love, perhaps he *is* good. We've all had a first love. We all know how wonderfully marvellous that made us feel in our teenage years. The surge of confidence it gave us when we showed off our boyfriend to our friends and everyone we knew. That's what Mazy needs now. More than anything, she needs to free herself from all the shackles that bind her and start to enjoy herself. Live, like the teenage girl she is. Live, like she hasn't done before.

Chapter 38

Mazy

He makes me feel good, I keep thinking, and I wonder what the hell he sees in me. *Of course, we have music in common. Must be that, really. What else? Or he must think I'm really popular and he wants someone well-liked by his side. If only he knew!*

It's fun and exciting at the beginning. Going out, dancing, clubbing. All new to me but still fun and exciting. It's amazing just to be together, chatting endlessly about anything under the sun. It's easy to confuse this idyllic happiness with love, especially when so young. I feel almost carefree for once; though this feeling, like always, does *not* last very long.

Ethan comes round to meet my family, after quite some time. I realise I can't let him into my room. I can't bring myself to open the door, touch the door knob without going through the eternal rituals. How do I keep all this from him? From sheer bliss, I see myself fall into the abyss, in a fraction of a second. This time from a high. I fret in an inexplicable frenzy, so bizarre to anyone's eyes. I enter into panic mode. Quick! I have to hide my despair. Ethan will notice. It gets harder and harder to put on a face in front of those I love. And the demons chuckle and gloat. I can hear them, almost even see them. The anxiety is stabbing me from all directions. It's overpowering. I need to get out, somehow. I need to breathe. I'm suffocating.

Ethan follows me. "Hey! What was all that about?" he quizzes. A question mark sits sceptically all over his face. I eye him, despondently. I can't bring myself to tell him right now. Not here, not now. It's not the right moment. Besides, where would I begin? And I wonder how long it will take him to flee; to be out of the picture for good.

We drive around for a while, till the old banger complains. Time to stop for a while, give the car a chance to cool down.

"It's the radiator again. Must tell Dad to look at it." Ethan checks it. "This will give us *all* a chance to cool down," he smiles wryly and gives my hand a squeeze.

The view of the bay is breathtaking. It's just lovely to be there and watch the magnificent sunset hide slowly on the horizon, leaving its orange trail behind. Like shadows, only these are ablaze. The sailing boats, barely a dot on an immense floor of blue, make their way, leisurely, to the pontoons. The calm before the storm, I sense glumly. A prelude to what's to come. I tilt my head back and I sigh, almost desperately, though it wasn't my intention to sound desperate.

There must be only, one small step from thoughts to actions. And so, without even expecting to, I pour my heart out to Ethan. Another person in less than six months. First my shrink, now Ethan. Almost a stranger. I risk having my secret out there. But the words cascade forcefully like rapids, once in flow, impossible to detain. Yet somehow, I don't care, and all because I think I'm falling in love.

Looking back, I know I never really fell in love with Ethan. It was more of a teenage crush than anything, at the beginning.

Later, I guess, all I do is use him selfishly, for reassurance, mainly. Not that I'm proud of it, in all honesty, but that's the way the ball rolls.

Chapter 39

Freya

There's no hoping for the best with Mazy. It's always the same. Just when I'm so absolutely thrilled for her, and so glad that Ethan has come into her life, everything starts to dissipate. Just when I'm so sure this relationship will do her a world of good, get her out and about and make her demons and monsters disappear, what happens? Earth calls me from my seventh heaven and I land headfirst with the most painful of thuds.

Ethan's first evening at home promises to be a warm, happy, comfortable, cosy, and I could go on, family get-together. Disappointing, I'm afraid, to say the least, is actually the outcome. I suppose, by now, I should be used to the fact that with Mazy, it's a never-ending tale of uncertainty. She's so unpredictable, or should I actually say predictable, because deep down, we've seen this behaviour far too often. Therefore, we all usually have an inner, niggling hunch about how things may suddenly twist.

One moment she's almost euphoric. The next is beyond everyone's understanding. We sit down and enjoy a lovely, cold buffet. Mum has excelled herself today. We talk awkwardly at times, at others, rather animatedly but all in all, the meal goes as well as can be expected, for any first meal with a 'stranger'. Even Ella deserves a positive mention. Her ever-dynamic charisma keeps the conversation alive. Mum and Dad relax.

They don't interrogate Ethan, as I imagine Mazy dreaded, and he seems comfortable enough.

Who would think that after dessert, our little reunion would turn sour for those present? I suppose Ethan wants to see Mazy's room. That's what triggers it, no doubt. Perhaps he asks her to show him around the house which she does, quite willingly, till it comes to her blessed sanctuary. That's when Mazy's face becomes a picture of anguish. I watch it turn from red to purple. She stumbles and hesitates and my heart skips a beat, or two, or three. She's on the verge of fainting. Next, she breathes unusually quickly, as if she were asphyxiating. Worried and in disbelief, I call out for Mum. I try to grab Mazy by the arm, or she'll fall. But a dismayed Mazy runs out of the house and disappears. Mum and I stand still as if turned to stone, unable to believe the unexpected turn the evening has taken.

We switch our bemused eyes hastily to Ethan and see his baffled face.

He runs after her and also disappears, leaving us agape. I suppose they have a long conversation ahead of them. I'm glad Ella sits in the lounge with her knees curled up on the sofa, idly flicking through the channels. So glad she misses this uneasy moment. Otherwise, she would have pestered Mazy to open the sanctuary door and that, undoubtedly, would have made her collapse.

Mum gives me the *"wretched sanctuary is going to be the death of Mazy"* look but I'm too tired and upset to say anything. Too tired to think straight, and more so to hope that what's just happened will surely have a positive outcome. Too tired to even pray. Especially when it always seems to be in vain.

Chapter 40

Sandy

I need some quiet time to myself. To hide away. Have no one disturb me. Is it too much to ask? Sometimes I feel bad complaining about our lives and everything that is happening to us. I shouldn't make a mountain out of a molehill. I know all this is a light cross to bear, compared to what other families go through. It makes me guilty to feel sorry for myself, so I quickly snap out of it and pretend my eyes are teary because the pollen is high. That's why it always seems that I have permeable skin that expels everything that falls on it, allowing me to keep going. It's not exactly like that, though. There's a lot I bottle inside. Not really wanting it to come to the surface, so as not to worry anyone unnecessarily.

Yet I can't stop worrying about Mazy, at times even excessively. I make myself distraught thinking about her future. What type of life will she lead? Will she be successful? Will she give up on herself? Should I raise my hopes? Shouldn't I? I'm so hopeful sometimes. Why is it then that I suddenly have second thoughts?

Freya and Ella occupy my mind as well, of course. I know they struggle, too, with their lives and with Mazy's situation. I'm aware each of them is concerned and care about Mazy in their own special ways. Bless them, my babies! They'll soon walk the world on their own. Like I did and like my brother, too.

With this rat-race of a life that we lead today, it is with much shame that I admit, I do not often think about my brother. I can't forget, though, that boy with tousled, dark brown hair who teased me constantly, until I too, got my own back. His cheeky, freckled face and mischievous hazel eyes gave him away, whenever there was trouble. He grew into a tall, fine, handsome man. Still with a roguish look about him, so adored by all the females who came in and out of his life. Ella reminds me a lot of him; though I hope she doesn't lose touch with her family, like he did.

James finishes his studies around 1976 and almost simultaneously, is successful in getting a job he applies for in Wales. Before he takes up his post as a civil engineer, he comes home to marry his ever-loving girlfriend, Joanne and together they settle in Cardiff. Later they immigrate to Australia. Once he takes off, he forgets everyone he leaves behind. I struggle to keep the communication going but it takes two to tango. There comes a day when I get tired of trying and give up.

Now that I'm reminiscing on the past, I realise how much time is wasted over stupid, insignificant things that mean nothing, yet can destroy a relationship, separating us more than all the miles that lie between us. I agree, it's both strange and sad. I know one day when I'm ready, I'll get around to sorting this out. I guess I shouldn't wait too long before taking action. I seem to be pretty good at thinking, not acting. Just lingering on it. And there's certainly no excuse for either of us to reach this shameful outcome. We'll regret it terribly someday, I know.

Chapter 41

Mazy

I take a glimpse, in between words, to observe Ethan's face. A breather, too, amid sips of water, for my mouth feels parched. I don't think he understands. Maybe I've frightened him. I've inundated him with my torments, so very unexpectedly and all at once. My heart sinks. I regret ever taking the plunge. Twinges of pain seize me slowly but sharply, making me almost wrench alarmingly. Still, he doesn't say a word. It's rather frustrating. Maybe he prefers to listen. I'm losing it now. I think I'm going nuts. Frenetically nuts.

"Well, say something, for Christ's sake! Have I scared you? Am I not the girl you thought I was? Hey! If you want to finish this before we go much further, I'll understand."

I gaze at him, long and slow. I can't make out what he's thinking. His eyes, small, of a peculiar grey, give nothing away. I observe his features. His nose and his mouth are bold and distinctive against a strong, angular face. I'm at the end of my tether now. I feel ashamed, mortified and embarrassed. I'll step out of the car. Run and keep running.

And suddenly there's no need. Ethan looks up, in search of my eyes and finally speaks. He says he doesn't care. He'll help me overcome my fears.

Together we can beat them.

"It happens," he says, "to many people. You are not alone," he affirms with unbelievable assurance. My heart skips a beat. I don't know whether to laugh or cry. My world is such a ferris wheel of inexorable emotions.

He holds me close. I feel appeased, yet I am trembling. He tells me he's astounded. Never guessed I suffered from a mental disorder. He never would have figured that my mind troubled me so.

"I know. I hide it as much as I can. It's my deep-rooted secret and that's the way I want it to stay," I confess, with uttermost surety. We talk endlessly. I seek reassurance and don't stop, until I hear the words I want to hear, cascading positively, from Ethan's mouth.

Back home, I can sense Mum and Freya are dying to ask me what's happened. Instead, they are cautious and don't probe. I bet they'll start prodding me tomorrow. They won't wait much longer. I check myself before I take it out on them. After all, I know they care and support me, no matter what. My demons react as I slouch on the sofa, completely exhausted. I was wondering how long it would take for them to do so. I wait for everyone to retire to their bedrooms, to embark on my never-ending rituals, before I step into my sanctuary. And then, that's when they start firing missiles. They hit their target right in the centre, as only *they* know how to.

Do you believe your boyfriend is telling you the truth? Honestly? Is that what you think? If you do, you are even more stupid than we imagined.

I cover my ears. I think I've had enough for one day. *Not they.*

Do you really think he's falling for you? Of all the girls he could have, do you think he'll want one, who is short of losing her wits? You'll end up alone, like always. You'll see.

I try to focus my attention on the sessions with Dr Barton. Everything he tells me to do in moments of panic; take deep breaths, write my feelings on paper, thinking about things that make me happy. I must centre my attention on what he's told me. I must! I must!

I pull my hair. I clench my teeth and bite the side of my forefinger in hopelessness.

Nothing works.

Chapter 42

Sandy

I return to the present. I don't want to continue reminiscing on the past. It saddens me and I don't want to feel low. I want to transmit happiness to all my crew. I often wonder how we'll get through the day. There are so many ups and downs to overcome. The longest obstacle race I've ever competed in, it seems. Ella tells me she's quitting school. I can't get over that. Freya seems like she's hit rock bottom. And Mazy, well, Mazy is just Mazy. But the cherry on the cake is now the new addition, I wasn't counting on, Ethan. Does he think I don't see how he has suddenly enveloped Mazy in his world? Oh! Yes! His house, his family, his relatives, his friends, his hobbies and everything that involves *him*. I don't know where all this leaves us because, quite frankly, I don't see us in the picture.

I hardly see Mazy now, just sporadically. When I do and I ask her about her relationship, she just shrugs. OK. I don't want to sound paranoid or act paranoid. I'm *not* jealous, either. Well, perhaps just a little. To be honest, I don't know how I feel. I guess I miss her. She doesn't even seek reassurance from me anymore.

"Mazy, how's things?" I start with calmness but then, I impulsively continue. "What's happening? Why are you always in his house? Don't you think it's too early in the relationship to be always with his family? You should be out and about, having fun with other friends your age."

In Defeat of Goliath

And I continue further. "What about the music? I don't see you go off to the band room as often. Don't let him take the music away from you, whatever you do!"

"We're fine, Mum. Honestly, everything's just fine," she adamantly retorts.

I know I must sound like a freak. It's hard to admit, but it's Mazy's time to fly. She's not a bird in a cage. I've always wanted to see her get up and go, so now that she's off, come on Sandy, let go of the reins, I convince myself. I daren't tell Eric about Ethan. He was the first to realise that, too many new things, were suddenly occurring in Mazy's life. He didn't exactly think them to be beneficial to her progress. I immediately disagreed. So, I'll let it go. Keep my feelings to myself. For now, at least.

I won't pressure Mazy anymore. I know it won't do anyone any good. After all, she's always been very sensible so I'll trust her better judgement where Ethan is concerned. Oh! Mothers! Mothers! Sometimes we are worse than everyone else. Speak for yourself, you may well say!

Freya seems very demoralised. I must give her all the encouragement I can. She's always there for everyone and now, it's certainly my turn to offer her support. I know, I'll take her out for a meal, just the two of us. Have a girlie afternoon together. Perhaps a little shop-till-we-drop spree. She'll like that, I'm sure. It'll lift her spirits and release some stress. God knows we need it!

And my thoughts return to Ella. *Whatever am I going to do with that girl?*

Chapter 43

Mazy

In every stage of our lives, there are good and bad memories. The good ones undoubtedly prevail. The bad ones are forced to vanish into thin air. I learn, with time and possibly the hard way, it's not always like that. Time does not wipe out the terror I endure in childhood and adolescence. I cannot eliminate the hardship that is so painful to remember. Like it never happened. Like a vaccine that eradicates whatever the ailment.

I research and research to find answers to endless questions, I desperately ask myself. I need to find out why me. Why is my mind so fearsome? Why am I held captive by thoughts and voices that echo uncontrollably through the winding passages of my mind? Call them demons, intruders, ogres, monsters, fiends. Take your pick. It's still *my* mind. It's still *me*. Am I the ogre, the demon, the fiend? Is my diagnosis correct? How can they tell? There are similarities between mental disorders. Is it OCD, is it Pure O? Are there traits of bipolar or schizophrenia? I know I'll lose it if I'm not careful.

I realise now, nothing is coincidental. We live through everything the universe plans for us. And we live it as we choose because that's the way it's meant to be. Every circumstance, however terrible, reinforces us. And it doesn't matter if we make mistakes along the way because that helps us to grow as a person. It enables us to overcome the physical or mental horror we face each day. It makes us wiser and enriches us with an awareness of the true meaning of life.

Music. Ethan. Work. University. And everything that comes after. Nothing is planned, certainly not by me. Yet, it unfolds before me in no time, like a red carpet for a celebrity. Only I'm no celebrity. I'm a lost being. A stray piece in the jigsaw of life that fits nowhere. And something tells me, I will be rolling like a stone that gathers no moss until I find where I belong.

Being with Ethan, if only for a short period in my life, is a great eye-opener for me. It paves the way and prepares me for things to come. Things I never imagined would become a reality. Like interacting with Ethan's family, to begin with. Learning to live with them. Total strangers, who I awkwardly meet one day and socialise with, the next. Who I visit regularly from then on, despite how difficult it is for me to do so. They don't have a clue about the infinite rituals I carry out in my head, to help me through those moments. Ordinary moments so perfectly normal for anyone. Yet so agonizingly hard for me.

I don't realise, then, the lesson I am about to learn. I do now. One of living with others. Of giving and taking. Of being unselfish, thoughtful and considerate. Those principles and values, I was religiously taught, since I could reason, I forget to apply to myself, as I grow older. I blame my disorder for that. It's easy to do. Say I am not in my right frame of mind. The perfect excuse.

Chapter 44

Eric

"It's just for a short while. I'll pick up in a year of two," Mazy declares unexpectedly after she announces that she has something important to tell us.

I can't believe what I'm hearing. I take a fleeting look at Sandy to see if she is aware of any of this. Certainly not. Her mouth is wide open, her eyes quizzical in a face totally perplexed.

A sabbatical year? It's got to be a joke! Surely Mazy won't quit school now that she's reaping the fruits of her tremendous efforts. And only God knows how very, very difficult those efforts have been, and continue to be for her. Her exam results are absolutely incredible. She could be accepted into any of the best universities there are.

"Mazy, what are you saying? You were so keen to go to university, how is it you have suddenly changed your mind?" Sandy is going berserk with this decision. She doesn't understand anything. I can't blame her. I'm not happy either.

She thinks it's Ethan's doing. Dragging her with him down under to wherever it is he's heading. Changing her future plans and ambitions which have been so very hard for Mazy to achieve. It's been a slow, bumpy ride to where we are today. I want to think that Mazy has a will of her own and that she can stand up for herself. Not be persuaded, in any way, to do something she hasn't really planned.

"I want to work for some time. I want to earn money. Enjoy a different experience. It'll be most challenging for me, don't you think?"

Sandy and I are speechless. Dumbfounded. Another bombshell, that's exploded in our faces, without prior warning. I suddenly see a Mazy incredibly sure of herself. Extremely sure of what she wants. Resolute and steadfast. We fill her in with the pros and cons. I doubt she listens. It's a tricky situation. Why? For anyone, perhaps, this situation is just a break, a short parenthesis. They resume their goals, without the slightest difficulty, when ready. But for Mazy, who can guarantee how she will be in two years' time? Who can tell how her powerful mind will react?

"What I really want is to tour the world, with guitar on my back. Sing out my life to the human race, shower them with my music, my lyrics. Maybe then, everyone will understand me and the mental pain, I bear heavily on my shoulders," she softly concludes. Her voice, though barely a whisper, lingers in the air, oppressing my throat, till I can hardly breathe. Penetrating my heart with an instant sadness, that's so distressing for anyone, and more so for any parent.

Once again, what do you do? Do you refuse? What are the chances that Mazy will fall further into depression? What are the chances that, this time, Mazy will not be able to resurge from the ashes of despair, and continue with the motivation that thrives in her now?

Regrettably, suicide is always buried in the deepest clefts of our thoughts. It's always there, that feeling, solitary, hidden, often forgotten, but there, always there. Like a tireless stalker, who never gives up and hides in the shadows. I shudder at the thought and wave it away from my mind, for it will ruin my day.

So, we give in. We accept Mazy's new quest, after careful consideration. We realise it's not such a bad idea after all. Work is a great learning experience. It'll do her good to be part of a team. She'll meet new people and possibly change her inflexible mindset.

For we realise she is lost and desperately needs to find her way.

Chapter 45

Ella

I hated those days. I remember them well. Hate is a strong word, I know, but I think I hated Mazy just as much, or more. Couldn't understand anything. Didn't have the time or the patience, either. After all, we were only kids. Later stepping into adolescence. So, all I wanted then was to have fun. And that particular day, I knew it wouldn't be long before the storm that had been brewing for a long time, finally broke out.

Ha! Mazy decides to take a year out of school and everything is fine. I mention to Mum that I don't want to continue in school either, and fireworks shoot from all directions. Nope! I'm not listening to anyone. Not this time. They can preach all they like and try to reason with me, but I refuse to accept this. I'm so mad and so fed up with the same situation, that I just don't know how I continue here. Well! Of course, I know. I don't have money, that's why I'm *still* here. That's the only thing that ties me to this place. And the reason I want to work, too. I'll move out as soon as I can. Freya knows my plan.

Poor Freya! I almost destroyed her, back then. She was everyone's comfort, spreading her soothing balm of words on all of us. Even Mum and Dad stood strong most of the time, thanks to her support. I was so livid, nearly always. I couldn't stand her taking sides.

I see Mazy in front of me and all I know is that I go for her, without the slightest bit of remorse. I grab hold of her hair and pull it as hard as I can, till I almost snatch a handful. Whilst Mazy yells in excruciating pain, I push her with all my might and knock her over the coffee table. It has a dimmed glass top which shatters in millions of shards, cutting into Mazy's arms, as her body plunges uncontrollably over it. I scream all sorts of abusive words at her. Words so offensive and insulting, I don't know how I drive Mazy to ultimate insanity, there and then. I continue, without shame or regret, firing from my mouth such foul language, even I am astounded at my capacity to hurt.

Mum and Dad dash in, puzzled, confused at the commotion. Their faces change instantly from sheer bewilderment to horror. Freya is there already, trying desperately to steer me away from the scene, urging me frantically to calm down. Hushing me, cautiously, for there is both fear and grief in her eyes. But I am beside myself with rage, with the anger I have slowly weaved all these years, till suddenly, one day, it fearlessly emerges. Without warning, without boundaries.

And Mazy? She lashes out too. Furious and revengeful, she vomits her resentment on me. A resentment she, too, has gradually loomed through time and now cannot be restrained. Dad intervenes, his eyes stern but streaked with inconceivable anguish. He knew one day we would explode but like this? This is possibly beyond his belief.

I never apologised, as I recall, but that was me, then. Quite a monster! Cold, arrogant and totally unsympathetic. And I continue to believe, at the time, that everything about Mazy is superfluous, like the cuts she suffered that day. What was I becoming? Freya kept asking me that over and over. She threatened never to speak to me again, if I didn't, at least, try to understand Mazy and accept her mental state of imbalance. Not her dramas or her quest for attention, as I truly believed Mazy's problems to be.

I realise now, that most of all, I blamed Mazy for what she doing to our family. The pain we endured, often silently. The uneasiness she bombarded us with, each day. The negativity she parachuted upon us, from one minute to the next. The fear of the unknown, *that* is what I actually dreaded and couldn't bring myself to understand. Or even explain how I felt to my family, for I thought they wouldn't listen. It would be *me* they wouldn't understand.

Chapter 46

Sandy

There are so many things I fear in life. So, I hope and pray. I scheme and dream. Each night, each day. From the moment I wake up, I want the day to go well. I want the same for my family. I want them free from harm, from evil or ill health. I want them to steer in the right direction, with no obstacles in their way. It's what everybody wants, isn't it? I want a family, united through thick and thin. I never had it as a child. I had parents so very, very independent, they went their separate ways. The word together did not form part of their vocabulary, and therefore, they did not know its meaning. They were not always loving or affectionate. More than often strict and severe and I grew up lonely, distant and somewhat distrusting. I thought it was normal.

I saw mothers hugging and kissing their children and I yearned for a taste of that love, that warmth and affection. It didn't seem to come to them in dribs and drabs. But I grew up without emotions, without fuss. A hot meal and a roof over my head, I was told was more than enough. So I didn't complain and continued my journey. For they were not bad, nor cruel in any way, just unemotional, inexpressive, firm to their beliefs. They mellowed as they got older. More loving and kind-hearted to my children than they ever were to me, or to James. Possibly, too, the reason why my brother took flight and never returned, not even to visit.

And now I have a family of my own, the one I dreamed about whilst growing up, I know not to follow their example. I shower my children with the love I went without. I tell them blood is thicker and though I know it's not always the case, I instil in them a sense of duty, care and responsibility for one another. They must look out for each other, come what may, I tell them.

Yet how ironic! You can take a horse to water, but you cannot make it drink. That's my Ella, the indomitable horse that will not quench its thirst, though many fountains be at hand. It's hard to accept that history repeats itself. And I see before me, my Mum, Aida, all over again. Only this time she's Ella. The similarity is daunting but there are differences, too. For Ella changes with people. She's everything everyone admires and wants to be. Why not with Mazy?

What we live through this day is beyond our wildest imagination. The abuse, till now, is always verbal. Eric and I cannot tolerate how this escalates, more and more. We profess our disapproval, our rejection of their attitude often enough, each time we see them getting out of hand. They mutter under their breath, they shrug and they seem not to care. Their indestructible pride is their worst enemy. It's hard to keep calm and in control. It may be best to fly off the handle. Give them a taste of their own medicine. Maybe then, they'll come to their senses. But they don't, no matter our patience and tolerance. No matter our self-control or lack of it, they don't change their feelings for one another. And what I fear and dread, occurs.

I see them so enraged that day, it's frightening. I'm chilled from head to toe. Frozen to the spot, for surely it's not my daughters here before me. I do not want to relive it in my mind, for it's a nightmare of the worst kind. A lifetime of devotion to our children, of implanting principles and values, of giving them our undivided attention, shoots out of the window in little less than a flash.

And the ache in our hearts is as repressive, as the burden of guilt we bear.

Chapter 47

Mazy

I hear Mum use her favourite phrases, often enough, as she speaks. Out of the frying pan and into the fire, is one that now comes to mind. For I jump from a great problem to an even greater one. Like a fragile grasshopper, that from leap to leap and in all innocence ends in the gecko's mouth. I may not be that innocent and they may think I'm crazy, but isn't Ella crazier than me? After all, I don't attack anyone and heaven knows how many times I'd like to discharge my accumulated wrath on more than a person. Instead, I check myself. It's enough having to render to my demons each time. Like I owe them my life, my whole being, my existence.

It's no big deal for Ella to fight me. She always admits, even to my face, she can't stand me. Only this time, she turns physical. I'm glad I hit back at her, too. Bring her down from her high horse. She'll think twice before she next lifts a finger against me.

Of course, once it's over, she doesn't stop to think how violent and aggressive she's become. It's over and it's out of her mind just like that. In the flutter of an eyelid. But not for me. For Ella doesn't hear the voices in my head, bellowing at their highest level. She doesn't hear them hollering, till my eardrums thump and throb wildly against my temples. And I lose the will to live.

She opened the door to your sanctuary. She has the key. She took your precious belongings away from you. She touched everything and exposed them to millions of germs. She left the window open. It rained last night. The rain gushed in and ruined everything in there. YOU'VE LOST EVERYTHING.

I sink further into myself. For the monstrous voices are cruel and heartless. As pitiless as can be. The rituals will never cease, for how else will I subdue my compulsions? I can't keep going otherwise.

The war of wars breaks out in the immense battlefield of my mind. Demons wrestle to rid me of strength and energy. To enforce their will on me, like they always do. They tell me I must check every corner of my room, and despite my exhaustion, I comply, almost robotically. I know, whoever can see me now will cringe at the sight and believe insanity has overpowered me. That there is no hope left for me.

I lose count of how many times I carry out the same ritual, over and over. I scrutinise each millimetre of the walls, drastically touching and feeling them, for the voices say they are damp. I continue till my arms ache and my hands are sore. I'm so confused, they make me believe they *are* wet from the rain. Yet, it hasn't even rained and I *know* that. In the midst of the mayhem, I hear my voice, distant, perhaps distorted, trying desperately to pacify the demons. They do not listen or pretend not to hear. And I recoil in sheer hopelessness.

I'm drained from all the rush of adrenaline. It leaves me powerless, immobile. As useless as a battery that can no longer be recharged. Even my soul sadly gives up and abandons my body. It can no longer withstand my tireless mind. I cringe in shame, for what more can a person lose? Even my dignity has been cruelly torn away from me.

Chapter 48

Freya

I lend my shoulder to this family for them to weep on. I have done so for as far as I can remember. It comes to me instinctively. All I want is to see them happy and at peace. I willingly offer them support and season them with words of comfort. For I know they need them. A sprinkle here, a sprinkle there. Like a spoonful of sugar that helps the medicine go down. Or so the song says. Though this time, the pain does not heal with sugar and spice. With kind words or positive actions.

I do not care about myself. My feelings, my emotions are nobody's business but my own. I hide them behind a beaming face, a pleasant smile. For I think I am strong and I can endure my pain and everyone else's. But I am wrong. Now, I am hurt, so very, very hurt. And I cannot forget the image in my mind of two sisters, reproaching each other, even their very existence. What we experienced that day leaves me totally defeated. Crushed to the very core of my inner being. My constant mediating between the two, since childhood and even before, for it seems I was born mature, suddenly seems worthless. A useless attempt. A waste of time, through all these years. I am stripped of all readiness to continue in my pledge to help, whoever. For I suddenly realise that nobody cares. Because they refuse to change their ways. Because they are too caught in the selfish webs of their lives.

So now, perhaps it's time I change, too. Think about myself. Place myself first. I wonder if I can. I know I must try and try hard. As otherwise, they'll continue to take me for granted. They'll assume I'll always be there for them, without failure, especially when the going gets rough. What a big mistake! In any case, have they ever been aware of *my* problems? Do they even ask themselves if I'm OK? If there is something worrying me? The answer, I'm afraid, is a big NO, a *no* much bigger than their own egoism. So, I tell myself why bother?

I've been disheartened now for a while. Have they even asked what's wrong with me? The truth is, they haven't even noticed. I know Mum has and has often tried to encourage me, but not Ella or Mazy. For once, I shall stand back. I will not intervene or be that hand that rocks the cradle. And if I don't know how to do that, I shall learn. Possibly the hard way, but I *shall* learn. *Definitely.* For I am sick and tired of their attitudes. And if they cannot appreciate my being there for them always, then, it's time to withdraw.

I do not feel hate or anger. Those feelings do not dwell in me. I just feel hurt. And with the hurt comes indifference. They may not stay for long. I do not know. I do not even know whether I'll retract everything I say now. For all I presently feel for them is pity.

Chapter 49

Mazy

It's boring and monotonous! Well, I can't lie. I wish I could say it's totally satisfying but it isn't. Not at all what I expected. Work is a whole new experience for me. Unfortunately, not one bit gratifying. Definitely, nothing I ever imagined. It's not challenging at all. It's so easy, I can do it with my eyes wide shut. But I suppose that's what any admin post generally is, particularly in a law firm. Tedious and dull. Most afternoons just drag on and I feel so unmotivated, I almost doze off.

I am pleasantly surprised by my colleagues, though. They are a great lot. Fun, chatty, bubbly. Even the line managers are welcoming and approachable. They include me in everything, whether work-related or not, they always want me to join in their plans. What a difference to school life!

I hide my disorder as best as I can. It isn't easy. I speak about music. My guitar playing. My songwriting abilities. I want to fit in. I want to transition in as smoothly as possible. No dramas. I don't want to stand out. They think I'm cool. I want it to stay that way. The problems start soon. Of course, how strange would that be if there weren't problems around me! They follow me wherever I go. Or maybe it's because I create them for myself. Who knows?

There are big, old heavy dossiers stacked on top of metal cabinets. The stacks reach the ceiling. They are transcribing old data into newly bespoken computer programmes and systems. Updating their records. No need, then, for those massive files. They ask me to bring them down. To get hold of ladders and climb to the top. I reluctantly reach for them. No big deal for anyone. But for a person like me, a real nightmare. I try to hide a dismayed face that suddenly reveals itself. The one I don't want anybody to see. For the dossiers are covered thickly in dust and grime from the years they've sat there, eyeing us from above.

I flinch in disgust, as I try to assemble them in sequential order, before carrying them down. But my demons attack straight away, deafening my colleagues' voices. And before I have a chance to budge the wretched files, they hit me where it hurts the most. Yet another blow below the belt. They taunt me now, making a mockery of the millions of germs I've managed to spread everywhere. They gloat, till common sense shuts down and rapidly greys all notions of logic. Immediately, thoughts escalate. They transport me to my room, where I see myself desperately cleaning walls and furniture in absolute fanaticism, for fear the germs that are now in my hands, conquer and rule.

I've got to wash my hands. They are so filthy, I'm about to throw up.

I cannot continue. I jump down from the ladder in such haste, I almost lose my balance and knock it down with me. I don't want to give the game away. I've been terribly cautious, so far, to avoid suspicions. To keep inquisitive eyes from staring at me. To avoid the humiliation of catching them glancing at each other, perplexed, puzzled. I've measured my words and my actions, too, so no one can notice any underlying issues. But not today. Today I give my colleagues a show of my true colours.

Damn! Damn! Damn! Explanations now to everyone.

It's what I dread the most, having to come up with ridiculous excuses to hide the demonic mind that tortures me in glee. I'll tell them some hideous insect startled me. At least that'll do for now. Tomorrow, I don't know what I'll say to sound convincing.

Chapter 50

Sandy

I know I'm still annoyed with Mazy and Ella. I can't forget the unbelievable pain they caused us. Poor Freya is still suffering the consequences. If they think I will let this go off lightly, they can think again. I turn a blind eye many a time. Perhaps it's the wrong decision but I do it just the same. Sometimes for the benefit of all. Other times, because it's not the right moment to impose my will, or make drastic changes. I don't want to become the ever-tireless, nagging Mum.

Yet, I can't help feeling a sense of pride when I see Mazy go off to work each day, looking so smart. So strong and adamant to continue with her life, despite the immense struggle, I know it takes her, just to get out of bed and face the day. And I park my annoyance to one side, rather reluctantly, because half of me is still very upset and disappointed.

I may be very lenient with Mazy, I know. But I don't want to lose her in any way. Not with her condition, her mental instability. Especially not now, at this crucial time of her life. Teens are at such an unstable age, in any case. I want her to believe that we are truly there for her, come what may. Even Ella. Yes! *Even Ella*! As unlikely as it may seem, given their appalling relationship, I still know Ella would be there for Mazy, against all odds. Ella doesn't even know it, but her heart goes a long, long way. *I know.*

A strange feeling hovers around me. One, I don't know how to explain. I have always been Mazy's confidante. I know she survives on her reassurance fix. And I have got used to being that person who gives her reassurance, each time she needs it. It's not supposed to be a good thing for her, so her psychiatrist affirms. She has to stop using people to pacify her mind. Instead, she has to rely more and more on her better judgement. Till she grows more confident each day. Yet who doesn't seek reassurance each time something worries us? Particularly when our self-esteem tumbles and crashes to our feet. When it's so hard to pick up the pieces. It's so easy then, to turn to someone you trust and soothe your mental pain away, through words of comfort.

Now it's Ethan she turns to. It's the normal thing to do. We all confide in our partners. I confide in Eric. Always have since day one. More than in anyone else. Yet it worries me that Ethan may not give her the sound advice she requires to progress. I don't want anything to be detrimental to her mental state. I must confess, at first, I felt like an old toy that's been thrown aside. Terribly used and consequently worn out, replaced by a new one. As simple as that. And *that* hurts. I want Mazy in my life and it scares me that she may stop talking to me about all the things we've always shared. Things, I know have helped her to move forward. I see her act now, often, as if we are invisible. I want to see and feel that we are present in Mazy's life.

I've reflected a lot on this matter. I haven't even shared it with anyone, for fear they'll jump to the wrong conclusions. Think I'm jealous, for instance. Tell me not to interfere. I honestly don't want to make hasty decisions, that may only end in more useless arguments. The last thing I want to do is cause unnecessary problems in their relationship. On the contrary, I *really* want them to be happy. Anything to help Mazy get mentally better is a positive move. So where does that leave me?

Once again, patience seems to be the key denominator in my life. It's what I turn to when everything else fails. Or when it's best to retreat in silence. When everything looks bleak and the future seems too overwhelming to even think of it, I resort to a loyal friend, by the name of patience. I tell myself that everything will be fine if only I'm patient. And I learn to wait. Didn't someone, somewhere, say that good things come to those who wait? I only hope he or she wasn't lying because waiting patiently is the story of my life.

Chapter 51

Freya

Here I go again, back to square one! Yes! I guess I can't change the way I am, no matter how I try. Once more, I am anxious about everyone and everything around me. My family means the world to me. I *can't* and *won't* turn my back on them, even if I try.

I'm glad I've snapped out of this feeling-sorry-for-myself attitude, that suddenly overwhelmed me so profoundly. I suppose, in the same way as I accept everyone the way they are, I too, have to accept myself as I am. And this is *me;* I'm everyone's guardian angel. I realise now, I can't change that. I will, however, start to think more about myself. I want to seriously think about my future. I've been giving some thought lately, to what I'd like to do, once I leave school. Working with children seems to occupy my mind more and more each day. Perhaps working in pre-school, as a learning support assistant, would be good.

I believe I have the appropriate qualities, a calm and helpful disposition, necessary to help children at this early stage of their educational development. The first rung of the ladder in their long, learning journey. I think that will give me tremendous job satisfaction. I wouldn't like to be in a job that is monotonous, nearly always carrying out the same dull routines. How perfectly boring would that be! Yuk! I'd hate that!

In Defeat of Goliath

Poor Mazy! I know that's what she's feeling at the moment. Her admin work is so uninteresting, that despite being recently promoted, she still finds her new tasks equally unsatisfying. I guess she's cut out for work that is much more challenging, motivating and demanding. Something that will, undoubtedly, keep her extraordinary brain ticking, good and strong.

Hope and excitement seemed to spark from her eyes, like firecrackers ablaze, when she decided, unexpectedly, to change her world over. To replace her world of studies with the world of work. I know she wants to be financially independent, at all costs. That's why she doesn't give much thought to the type of job she chooses. Definitely, she won't stay in that lawyer's firm for long. Her anxiety won't let her. I realise she wants to earn money straight away to be able to fulfil her dreams. She wants to be a singer/song writer. It's a hard road to hit. I'm sure, though, if she makes it, she'll be one of a kind. Her voice, so harmonious, is absolutely incredible. As incredible as the fact that she adores rock. Seeing Mazy up on stage is the last thing that would have entered my mind. She certainly has caught us all by surprise.

We've been chatting lately about another possible change. Mazy needs to further her studies. Go off to university. Set herself other goals and objectives, a plan B. Have something up her sleeve, should her singing career fail. In any case, she can sing and write music in between classes. At university, everything is easier. More flexible. And she could possibly earn some money as well, jamming when she's free.

But she is still so lost. Doesn't really know which way to go. That's why I feel bad about turning my back on her. I've got to continue as always. Giving her moral support and encouraging her when she is low. I need to help her find her way, even though I still haven't, in all honesty, found mine.

Chapter 52

Mazy

I'm being totally unfair to Ethan. I know he doesn't deserve to be used, like I'm using him, to satisfy my unquenchable need for reassurance. I don't know why I do this, really. It's like a drug I'm addicted to. I realise I just can't go on, without hearing the words I want to hear. And they've *got* to come, now, from Ethan's mouth. Not from anyone else's. Perhaps if I smoked or drank more alcohol, I wouldn't have this insatiable desire to seek reassurance from him. Because I'd have something to turn to, to rely on when hope is but an impossible dream.

It's sickening, I know. It makes me feel so small and insignificant, it's pathetic. I don't need this. So why do I do it? Deep down I know. I divulge my secrets to Ethan and he becomes my shoulder to cry on. I shower him constantly with my ever-growing combo of worries, fears and insecurities. A dangerous cocktail that will someday explode in my face. But my anxiety is tempered by his words of comfort and encouragement. They give me hope and serenity, if only momentarily. So, I let the bond grow. The feeling of dependency is so very deplorable. It's enslaving. I go to him like iron to a magnet. Like oxygen for breathing. Nothing else. First, my Mum, now Ethan.

I've asked Dr Barton about this, often enough. I tried to use him, too, for reassurance. But he won't fall into my trap like Mum and Ethan. On the contrary. He wants me to accept myself for who I am. He wants me to believe in myself. To value my thoughts, my feelings, my opinions. To value myself as a person.

"Think highly of yourself. You have many talents that you submissively suppress. Don't bury them anymore, let them come to the surface. Don't be so hard on yourself," he tells me, each time.

The gush of confidence he gives me does not last for long. The good things just don't seem to stay with me. The following day, I wake up with the emptiness of heart and the vagueness of mind, that so shadow me for as long as I can remember. It's then I have to seek that reassurance, I can't even offer myself. Those words of comfort can make me stand tall and not snap like a twig from a tree. I so want to stand tall, like I do on any stage with any song that I can sing.

I feel I've been stagnant for a good while now. Part of me wants to move on to greener pastures. I can't play the part at work anymore, for I know I will collapse. My brain feels totally useless. I may take Freya up on her suggestion about going to university, I mean. Recently, I've been reflecting deeply on my future and studying psychology seems to me like a great idea. It's something I am presently contemplating through and through if only to better understand that maze of a mind that dwells in me. Maybe then I can overcome my demons. At the moment, I'm afraid *they* are winning and I can't let them keep scoring. Reason why I prefer to quit work now before something shameful occurs and my colleagues remember me for all the wrong reasons. Not for efficiency, competence or capability but for insanity.

But who can understand how I feel, when I can't even understand myself? Most of the time, I would like to run away and hide. Live like a hermit. I wouldn't need to be on the edge then, as I am now. For there would be nobody around to judge me. No farce, no masquerade, no false explanations to anyone. A great relief to a troubled mind, a fatigued body, an aching heart, a lost and weeping soul.

Chapter 53

Ella

Hey! What's new? Funnily enough, they've let me in on the latest. I hear from Freya, Mazy may be leaving us for a while. Off to university, I gather. Can't say I'm sorry she's leaving. In fact, what a relief! For the next three or four years, we'll have a break from our amazing Mazy. Can't wait, really. Only see her during hols, no doubt.

Mum and Dad are chuffed, too, over Mazy's decision. They were so worried that Mazy wouldn't be able to pick up her studies, where she left them. Good job her medication must be doing some good. Slowly but surely, it must be kicking in. Otherwise, Mazy would be far too void of motivation or the decision to embark on any new projects.

She worked for over two years. That's quite an achievement, I must say. It must have been quite a battle for her, trying to hide her disorder from her colleagues. I don't know how, but she did it. In the same way, I know, she can achieve anything she sets her mind to. That's why I am more convinced with each passing day, that Mazy does not suffer from mental issues. All she has ever wanted and sought is attention. To this day, still, if she doesn't get her fair share of it, she blows things out of proportion by dramatising everything. Attention and reassurance *have* to be the dish of the day, otherwise, nothing else matters.

If everyone listened to me like they listen to good old Mazy, I'm sure she would have snapped out of such a complicated attitude, that has so characterised her all these years. I would have helped her find friends, mix in entertaining circles and enjoy the many summers she spent, cooped up on her own.

I only hope that she doesn't create more problems for herself, than are absolutely necessary, *if* and *when* she goes to university. She'll certainly need friends there. Good ones too, whom she can trust and share accommodation with. *That* will undoubtedly be the greatest challenge yet to come. Knowing that her belongings are within easy reach of others, will be the utmost struggle of struggles for her. I sincerely hope she doesn't start to isolate herself from the very moment she arrives. If she doesn't mingle with other students from day one, then everything will be so much harder for her. In the beginning, everybody is eager to make friends and find their niche, where they are comfortable. Once the circles are formed, it's much more difficult to fit in.

It'll be great if she starts singing and playing as soon as possible. That would be a good way to meet other students, particularly those interested in music, like herself. Maybe she will form a band. There are many opportunities for students who are gifted in the arts. So, I sincerely hope she jumps on the train, this time.

Pity I don't have the brains to further my studies, if not I would definitely revolutionise the whole university, plus its campus, by partying till dead. Every day would be a killer, for I would ensure we'd all have a whale of a time. Students would just love being around me because fun, entertainment *and booze*, would surely be guaranteed. I may consider not leaving school after all. Now that Mazy will not be around for a while, it may not be that bad staying at home. So, who needs to work then and earn money? Or miss school holidays? Even miss a lie-in most mornings, after wild night outs?

Certainly not me!

Chapter 54

Sandy

I look around and see two bulging suitcases propped up against her bedroom wall, ready and waiting. It sinks in then. Mazy is leaving us. New future targets await her. Again, that bitter-sweet feeling strikes unremorsefully. And I don't know whether to cry or heave a sigh of relief. The obstacle race of our lives has finally got us to this point, which I hope, is of no return.

Mazy's decision to study psychology is well accepted. From then on, it's a mad commotion of conniving plans, which are simultaneously ravelled and unravelled, like yarn from a woolly jumper. Exciting times, though often stressful, take over our lives, almost instantly. But then, everything Mazy does enwraps us always in its entirety.

A thorough and extensive research of universities continues. I enjoy seeing Mazy buzzing with motivation. Stimulated to the core, to the very lining of her mind and beyond. I cross my fingers vehemently so that nothing can trespass that fine line where incentive, enthusiasm and encouragement now reside. Mazy applies to various universities throughout the United Kingdom, tirelessly trying to obtain as much information on psychology as possible. Some teach psychology to very high standards, particularly the 'red-brick' universities, and these require an even higher pass rate to achieve entrance.

"What about your music, Mazy?" Freya queries, "I thought you might want to study music performance and management, for example."

"This will be my plan B, Freya, just as you suggested," Mazy admits, steadfastly. "When I graduate from university, I'll centre my efforts on promoting my music. If this takes me nowhere, then I'll start a career in clinical psychology or as a lecturer in some college or even as a counsellor. Knowing what I go through with my OCD or this Pure O business, I can certainly give good advice to any one suffering the same disorder. No one better than me to understand those problems!"

Finally, she decides on a 'red brick' university, situated towards the North West of England. This university has recently been refurbished to meet the latest mandated standards of modern, state-of-the-art development, catering for a diverse range of student requisites. Plus, the main thing, it teaches psychology to the highest of standards.

Mazy is delighted and enthusiastically shows us the on-line prospectus, navigating through the extended halls of residence, the various spacious lecture rooms, the modernised science lab and the contemporary music room. A well-equipped gymnasium follows, together with a large indoor swimming-pool. Tennis courts, football pitches, a lunch hall that could run wild horses and endless other areas seem absolutely brilliant. The university campus boasts peaceful, eco-friendly gardens with magnificent views, so all in all, I can understand why Mazy is so excited.

"I'm so proud of you," I can't help but hug Mazy warmly. "I admire how sensible you are, Mazy, and that despite your worst moments, you are still able to keep your head above the water. Never stop swimming strongly against the tide, against all adversities. Don't forget the other side is always there, waiting for you to fulfil your aspired dreams."

Outride the demons, I pray with fervour. Let this be another turning point in your life. One that you can look up to with pride and confidence, acknowledging that when constant perseverance prevails, despite whatever impediment, nothing is impossible. No milestones are unachievable in today's world. Everyone has a place and a purpose whilst we are here, no matter the race or creed, disability or capability.

And Mazy, dearest, you are no different!

Part Three

Chapter 55

Mazy

I can't believe I'm actually turning my life around. I still don't know how. I mean, going to university may not present a problem for most, other than economically, perhaps, but for me, it's such a gigantic leap. Two years ago, I panicked terribly. I quit studying. Took a sabbatical year that turned into two. Couldn't face the imminent future. Decided to work instead. I cannot say it was the wrong decision. No, not really.

Work is good at the beginning. The tasks are mind-numbing though, to say the least, but mixing with colleagues is such a positive experience. It's a relief to know they also take to me, from day one. I never felt like this in school. So at ease. I should have opened up to them. Let them know about my disorder. Be truthful, for once. I guess I'm too much of a coward.

I'm glad I'm picking up my studies from where I left them. I do so much sooner than I anticipate, completing them successfully, to my entire satisfaction. This is a massive struggle because, whilst I try to juggle as many new things in life, as my mind permits, my relationship with Ethan, runs stale. It seems inevitable. I only use him as a friend. There's affection but not love. Impossible to continue. I'm glad it's over before we say things that really hurt us, that really hurt our families, too. So we go our separate ways, without dramas. That's good enough for me. I realise everything that has happened in my life so far, is actually positive. It paves the way for those greener pastures, I keep talking about.

It takes forever to sort out arrangements for university. The familiarisation visit is fantastic and reinforces further, my intentions to study psychology, if ever there were any doubts. I'm so busy, I just can't afford to hear the voices right now, and I battle to deafen them, lest they shatter my plans. But they are there, amidst the havoc trying to surface in whichever way possible.

The grant won't come through, they taunt, just to make me despair.

But it does. My grant is approved and here I am, onward bound on a train heading for North East England, with a degree in psychology to obtain as an objective. My greatest challenge is yet to come. I clutch my baggage, my laptop and my guitar like there is no tomorrow. Like my life depends on it. I cannot lose them. Nobody can steal them. I'm far too vigilant.

It starts to rain, first gently, then forcefully. Shit! Shit! Shit! My belongings are getting wet, as I wait for a taxi to take me to the halls of residence. I begin to have doubts. What the hell am I doing here? I should have done my degree on-line. This is too great a challenge for me. I doubt I'll be able to cope. I need to get a hold of myself before I lose control.

It's a new start, I tell myself. *The one you've been waiting for. The break, you've so yearned for, when mentally paralysed. You can't blow it now.* Am I reassuring myself, again? Yes, I answer my inner self.

Yes, I ask you, the 'me inside of me', when nobody else can reassure me, I turn to you.

I fumble in my coat pockets for tissues to dry my laptop-cover but my fingers are useless, in a hand that trembles incessantly. I'm drenched to the bone, too. I eye myself in dismay. And when I pay the taxi driver at the end of a tantalizing journey, I'm so giddy with nerves, I can't blame him for eying me perplexed. He probably suspects I've surpassed my alcohol limit. Little does he know!

I finally stumble into the halls. Surprisingly, still in one piece. All at once, I'm totally blown away by what I see. Thousands of students, from all walks of life, with as many bags as myself, are chitchatting animatedly in the grand reception hall. They await room allocation, or so I'm told by the receptionist.

First impressions are so overwhelming. So many people in one place make me uneasy. They turn their eyes on me. God! My insecurities kick in instantly. I want so badly to be swallowed up but the floor doesn't crumble before me, unfortunately, and everyone observes me. I take one long, deep breath and with guitar on back so that my passion for music does not go unnoticed, I make a tremendous effort to mingle with the crowds. I'm half excited, half shaky, half dazed, half not knowing what the hell I'm doing. I make various, futile attempts to find music enthusiasts, at least, to share a common interest.

If anything, I know I look cool with my guitar slung casually over my shoulder. It boosts my self-esteem and it's a cunning way of generating conversation. Something I've always found so difficult. I step back a little, to watch them. I like to people-watch. I'm able to learn so much about everyone just by studying them, whilst they are oblivious to being scrutinised. Their body language reveals more than they will ever admit. Perhaps studying psychology is going to be a piece of cake. Pity I can't understand my own mind.

And just before an invasive thought, regarding my bags, plagues the contours of my brain, I hear a friendly, high-pitched voice, approach me from behind. I turn around, ever so curious. I'm glad someone has taken a gamble on me.

"Hi there, who may you be with guitar on back? Don't tell me - hush - you are in a rock band, right? Your pale skin, dark hair and black gear tell me you are rock mad. Eh! Let's see, not into heavy metal though. Something softer, like Blink 182 perhaps?"

I'm taken aback. Who is this? Some kind of clairvoyant, I wonder.

"Two out of three, good guessing. Am I so predictable? I was hoping to be a bit more mysterious," I grin, pretending to sound as confident as can be. "Hi, I'm Mazy, by the way, and yes, I'm rock mad and I'm Blink 182's number one fan. I used to be in a band. Now I go solo. I write my own music and lyrics," I add, glad to find someone who enjoys my type of music.

"When will we see you perform then? You can join Band Soc. Anyone told you about it yet? Oops! Sorry, I'm Kelly and I'm Blink 182's second fan *if* you are their number one! I think we are in the same corridor."

"Oh! That's great then. And yes, I'll be glad to join Band Soc. I'll need to find out more about it. So, what are you studying then?"

"Psychology," Kelly confirms, with what seems to me, little or no enthusiasm whatsoever.

"No kidding, so am I," I admit, with at least more oomph than my newly-found neighbour.

I heave a sigh of relief, for now, the ice is broken and the first day is almost done.

Chapter 56

Sandy

The years in university are the greatest trial of endurance Mazy faces since she has been able to reason. If she can get through this, I think, she can get through anything. She inundates me with stories of freshers' week. Of joining Band Soc. She'll perform soon, she assures. And I'm delighted. There's Kelly, a neighbour, I gather. Her classes, they are just as she imagined them to be. Her tutors are all so very helpful, in particular, a Mr Chan, but he is so demanding. Too much to take in all at once. But I don't want her to stop. It fills me with such gratifying satisfaction.

The harder times I dread, come later, as I knew they would. The pressure and stress that studies place on anyone, are doubly felt by Mazy. Strict deadlines to meet, nerve-wracking exams that drive her to the limit, hours and hours of being buried in books, ruthlessly take their toll. It's then that she hits the temples of her head with fisted hands, in a terrifying act of desperation. It's when blood trickles fearfully down her nose and panic strikes, unsympathetically. But why? Why inflict physical pain, when there is already, so much mental agony? Is it because her mind is so fatigued, it is about to give up on her? Is she totally burned out? Perhaps, there is no further room in her mind. It's so very dwelled already and therefore impossible to retain all the psychological jargon, she has to learn. I imagine it's a culmination of everything, really.

It's then, too, when she phones or Skype's, almost hysterically, at erratic times, to seek as ever, her dose of reassurance. Maybe at four in the morning, maybe at five. Any time, during the day or night. There's no Ethan now in the picture, so it's back to me for reassurance. That's when she confesses how she cannot juggle different priorities, with the same deadlines for delivery. And as always, I try to calm her. I have that dose of reassurance ready and waiting to placate her troubled state of mind. I tell her how to make the best use of her time.

"Remember, Mazy, when you used to perform, study, and sit for exams? You managed then and you'll manage now," I desperately try to convince her. I only pray that she listens to me, instead of her demons. "Tell your tutors, Mazy," I advise, hiding as best I can, my extreme anxiety. "You can't go through this on your own. They'll help you like they help others in similar situations. Don't think you are the only student there with a mental disorder. There must be others," I try frantically, to plead with her.

"I don't want special treatment," she retorts abruptly. "This is something I've got to achieve, without concessions of any kind."

I try to sound as understanding as can be. I only hope my broken voice does not give me away. "You are exhausted, Mazy. Try to get some sleep. Things will not be as bleak tomorrow," I whisper, every time, day or night.

I sigh forlornly when she hangs up. I can't think why those invasive enemies never relinquish their mighty grasp on her, though try as she may, to struggle free. I do want to believe that, heartless and unyielding as they are, they are not yet conquerors. The battle is neither won nor over. No, *definitely* not. Those invaders will one day be defeated, I know. Mazy is like the fragile flower, that somehow blooms, no matter the inclement weather.

With each new experience, however excruciating, Mazy will learn to dethrone her demons. From the front line, they'll settle inaudibly behind the ranks, till they are nothing but history. The journey is far too long. We accompany her along the way, in proximity and at a distance. For we are always there for her. To listen and advise, whenever necessary.

Now she's on her own, living through rough times, though these are also positive and rewarding years. Years she'll always treasure and remember, for they help to reconstruct foundations that are on the verge of collapse. It's what catapults her to independence and enables her to emancipate later on in life, without fear or hesitation.

Chapter 57

Mazy

I enquire about Band Soc the very next day. I am invited to attend and if interested, to join. The university boasts an exclusive band society for students who are interested in music. It doesn't matter if you are a performer or simply just enjoy listening to music. All are welcome. The genre is pretty diverse, too. I'm so relieved by that. I hate being restricted in music. There are enough limitations in my life, already. Music is freedom. It's communication. It's bridging absolutely everything, creed, race and ideologies of any kind, with meaningful lyrics and rhythm. Music has no frontiers. And I so want to create songs that heal; songs that will stay wedged in the memory of generations to come.

But I cannot forget I have a mission. I have to come face to face with my disorder. I really have to confront my demons, never best said. I need desperately to learn and understand brain function, to enable me to understand *my own* brain malfunction. I know I cannot steer away from my objectives, though music will give me a break, a breather. I need that desperately, too.

"Hi there! Welcome to Band Soc." A friendly-looking, young man, greets me with certain, undeniable eagerness. He catches me admiring the grand music hall in absolute awe and smiles. "We all feel that way when we first step in here," he grins amusedly. "I'm John Hayward, the university's music co-ordinator."

"Hi, I'm Mazy and would certainly like to join Band Soc," I acknowledge, as I extend my hand to shake John's. His warm smile is his best feature. I just wish I could smile more often. Instead, more often than not, I frown and scowl. I guess that's what makes him look so young, plus the fact that he is tall and slim.

I eye him more closely, yet discretely and notice that John Hayward has thinning, reddish hair and pale skin, that looks like it would burn after five minutes in the sun.

"You play acoustic?" He seems direct, urging me to play, as he ushers me towards the stage. "You sing, too?" he continues. No time to waste, apparently, I gather.

"Yes, I sing and play the guitar, both acoustic and electric," I confirm, hoping he is impressed.

I gaze at the stage with the great respect it deserves. I can't fool myself. It scares me. It's much bigger than any I've performed on before, and that makes my stomach turn. It's complete, too, with high-powered amplifiers and classy sound systems, not even I have seen before. Quite awesome, I admit. I note a classical piano with little or none of its grandeur left, tucked away in a corner. It's definitely seen better days, though it must still be in use. A modern keyboard, however, sits on a stand in a more privileged position. It must think the old piano is of no competition.

"Sounds promising. Go on, get on stage, let me see you perform. We desperately need people to perform for freshers' week and that's next week."

"Oh! I wasn't counting on performing just now. I mean, I don't have anything prepared," I hesitate, rather taken aback by John's insistence.

"You know any covers you can sing?" he quizzes, trying not to sound like he's at the end of his tether. I suppose it's stressful, trying to organise all the musical events, for such an important week. "If you are good, I'll just book you," he concludes.

I heave my guitar carefully onto the stage and run up the steps. I check thoroughly the amps and microphones. I'm conscious I may be taking too long and John is watching, by now impatiently. I know because his forehead seems shiny and it's not from the lighting. And then, without further thought or realisation, I hear myself strum the chords and intone one of my favourite covers.

I suddenly come alive on stage. It doesn't take me much effort once I start. I'm miraculously transformed. John stops immediately to listen. For a moment he thinks the real singer is on stage, not someone totally unknown, singing a cover.

"*If I could, then I would...*" I try my hardest to project my voice. I expel the words, utterly heartfelt, till they resonate freely throughout the hall and beyond. Like a silver bullet shot from a .38. If only I could expel my demons in the same way, I contemplate sadly, as I battle to focus on the lyrics.

I'm oblivious to the large crowd that gathers in the doorway and pushes their way in to hear me sing. I'm gobsmacked at the cheer when I finish.

John stares at me intently, with eyes that are about to pop out of his face. "Wow! Wow! Wow!" is all he seems able to say. "Amazing! Absolutely amazing! Listen Mazy, you make sure you make no commitments next week because you are booked for Freshers' Week, every evening from 10:00 pm till late. You hear me?" John could hardly believe his luck. "Where have you been hiding all this time? You know, you have saved me! I was looking for someone like you and here you are, right in front of me."

What a marvellous feeling! This is how I want to feel - *always*.

And the voices? Where do they go? They go nowhere, for they make themselves heard before I can assimilate what has just happened.

"Be careful of the crowds," they scorn in malice. *"Don't let them touch your guitar. Put it away, safely in its cover. Quick, do it before they approach you."*

Almost mechanically, I turn my back on those who beckon to me in admiration and rapidly, I shove my guitar in its cover. Safe from dirty, grimy fingers that may dare touch its lovely brown enamelled body, against a sleek, glossy centre. I'm mortified once more, for my reactions are now almost robotic. It's as if I'm programmed by some hypothetical alien, and have no control over my actions.

Kelly is there amidst the crowd and my paranoia kicks in. *Has she noticed what I've just done?* I wonder, in absolute anguish. *Have they all observed my weird behaviour? Whatever are they thinking?*

I make every effort to dissimulate, with the minimum will and strength that remains in me. A plastic smile falls back on my face, yet again.

Kelly can't hold back her excitement. She isn't alone. New friends, recently acquired, accompany her. Becky, her partner Will and Josie, introduce themselves. They are full of praise for my performance. I try to keep my composure and finally, manage to breathe serenely, for I do believe they have not noticed. An injection of confidence zooms, with the speed of lightning, through every fibre of my body. I wish *that* confidence would stay within me. I don't want this wonderful feeling to evaporate tomorrow, like droplets of rain, as I know it will.

Chapter 58

Freya

The years roll quickly by, whilst Mazy is away. I grow up just as quickly, and my life changes drastically. I understand perfectly now, Mazy's decision to park her studies and start to work. I unexpectedly feel the same way and though I always want to become a pre-school teacher, I give up one day, out of the blue. Studying no longer motivates me, and despite my mother's endeavour to steer me in what she considers to be 'the right direction', I unwaveringly take another route.

I decide to work in administration for a leading and rapidly expanding organisation. It's a demanding job with good prospects for training and promotion. It provides me with the professional satisfaction and the financial independence, I seek. It isn't long before I reap the benefits. My social life spirals wildly, as a result. I lift my foot off the brakes for once in my life and stop being the mature creature, I have always been. I park aside that sensible me and start to enjoy life to the fullest. I'm suddenly the young adult I needed to be. Drinks after work, partying weekends, new funky clothes to show off to friends, new car to hit the road, become the reality I always yearned for.

I feel carefree, cheerful. Even popular. No one to worry about anymore. No one to nurture. No one's burden to carry. I've had enough. Mazy is mentally shackled, but I too, have been totally constrained by my endeavour to keep my family together. Now it's my time to get out there and enjoy myself, as much as possible.

I meet Graham, not long after. Graham Duncan. Mum is shocked to hear he is thirteen years older than me. But who cares what anyone thinks? Who pays heed to advice when it comes to love? As always alleged, love is blind and has no boundaries. It probably isn't love at first sight, but the spark is there, right from the start. And the spark grows more and more with each passing day. I learn everything about him. I like his looks, his slight build, his receding blonde hairline and his boundless energy, so I don't listen to the constant 'what do you see in him?' comments from others. I enjoy being with him. I enjoy how he treats me at the beginning. And when we are both ready to live together, I don't hesitate in moving in with him. End of story.

These are good years of fun and enjoyment. I welcome the break from being at the edge of the precipice almost every day. It gives me a much-earned respite from arguments, from mediating, nearly always.

I keep in touch with Mazy and comment on how our lives suddenly change. I see her frequently during holidays and admire how she keeps on going. She meets Graham and confirms her approval. I am pleased, though, of course, she only knows him superficially. In all honesty, everything now takes second place in my new list of priorities. I don't listen to anyone, not even to Mum, who tirelessly begs me not to move in with 'this guy'.

"Get to know him first, Freya," I remember how she almost wailed desperately. "Don't rush into anything. You are only seventeen, he's already thirty-one. He'll tie you down. You are living now. Continue to do so; enjoy yourself. There's so much time later to make commitments."

I just wish one of those priorities on that list had been to listen to Mum's wise words, that day. I just wish I knew then what I know now. I wish I could turn the clock back and annul, totally, everything that occurred in my life for the eleven years that followed. How living with a narcissist, a sociopath and a psychopath, all in one, changed me and the only good thing that came out of all the mental torture I endured, were my two precious children, Sophie and Colin, who helped me survive through my darkest hours.

But then, that's another story.

Chapter 59

Mazy

Peaks and troughs. I wonder if this is the best way to describe the emotional instability, I experience throughout those years. An importunate, zig-zag pattern of highs and lows, that so naturally emerge from within, without resilience. They are an eye-opener at all costs. The constant checking rituals become a nightmarish trauma, that almost lead me to the point of collapse. Time becomes my worst enemy, as I helplessly surrender to my insatiable compulsions. I hear the tick-tock of each passing minute with immeasurable agony and impotence, whilst I lie captive of a mind, that strips me of all power and will.

I want to squeeze time in a bottle and tighten the top but it defiantly refuses to be restrained and escapes through my fingers. And when I sit the exams, my mind is so trapped, it will not register the time I needlessly waste, checking every word, every answer I tremulously write. My thoughts are bolted, forbidding my hand to continue. I look around and see everyone confidently page-turning and in progress, whilst I swim in conflict against the tide. And time continues to defy me, as do my demons. I steal a frightful glance at the clock as it strikes mercilessly, alongside the failing beat of my heart. I cringe in shameful despair. I pick up whatever dwindling strength I have left and continue in haste, for now, time is almost up.

It's when I erroneously decide to stop taking my medication, too. Another trough I crawl through blindly amid the mayhem. I research extensively the effect, nutrition has on mental disorders. I resolve to eat healthily there and then. No need to take long-term medication, in that case. Such an extremist, I doubt I know who I am. I shoot downhill as a result, right into the face of depression. How can I be so incredibly lost?

It's when I start to isolate and refuse to socialise with anyone, just when I was beginning to unwind gradually and enjoy a few beers with the gang. I stop going to pubs, where until now, I have even jammed to the amazement of all. They tell me I'm good. I have potential. They want more. Now I can't bring myself to believe them. I refuse to attend Band Soc. No further performances. I give no reasons, no excuses. I leave everyone with a thirst for more. No wonder they shrug their shoulders, curious and perplexed.

I live in shared accommodation. How difficult is that? My housemates are aspiring psychologists, who can easily pick up on strange behaviours. No one is stupid. They pick up the signals. It's even harder to avoid the inevitable questions. Again, the exchange of fleeting glances, baffled and bewildered. And all I want to do is vanish, never to be found.

I should let the world know what is wrong with me. Why the torture of keeping it hushed, when practically everyone can assume what is obvious? But logic does not dwell within me. Instead, I let everyone see me at my worst. I allow the bizarre creature that lies within me to escape to the surface, as I always do. And all for no sound reason, other than to create more unnecessary torment for myself.

Chapter 60

Ella

"If I don't do things now that I am young, when will I do them? When I'm tied down with a family and other commitments?" I often retort, irritably. I hate having to justify myself to everyone, each time they disapprove of any rushed decision I take. It's my life and I don't want it to stay dormant, or feel ensnared in a no-win situation. I want changes that motivate me and trigger my adrenalin to the highest of peaks.

I am the same carefree spirit I was as a child. I plunge headfirst into any situation, without fear of consequences. I think everyone resents me for that as well as for so many other things. Nothing can be worse than being unhappy, so I don't hesitate to put a stop to that, whenever the case arises. I know I go in and out of jobs, without the slightest bit of regret. The moment they stop stimulating my senses, I quit and move on.

"It will pave the way for something better," I say to others, as they stare dumbfounded and in dismay. I don't care what they think, for I know how to play the game of life. I know how to move the markers strategically in life's complex game, despite everyone's scepticism. And when I see an opportunity dangling before my very eyes, I seize it before someone else grabs it selfishly and never lets it go.

Like Freya, my life changes, too, from the moment I meet Gerry. We are two live wires as if fused by an electromagnetic force of the highest voltage. We are unstoppable. Together it's as if fate is on our side. Like we hold the winning ticket and we can overcome the obstacles that life hurls in our way. I never believed or even dreamed of meeting my 'other half'. Strangely enough, I do. No other relationship has ever lasted, at least, not much longer than I could keep a job. It strikes me how everything in my life makes a grand, dynamic entrance and then, without the slightest bit of anticipation, vanishes just as quickly as it appears. But that changes one day, the day Gerry comes and stays.

I enjoy the night life. Crammed discos, bursting at the seams, reeking of booze and sweat. Flashing lights that blind me. Music blaring at the twist of every bend. I dance wildly to the beat. I feel the adrenalin pump, uncontrollably, through my veins. The pungent smell of booze lingers on my breath, in my clothes, in the atmosphere. I love every bit of it and wouldn't change a thing. It's where and how I meet Gerry at the pinnacle of the night when the fun is at its highest.

I can't really recall how it all happened. He is dancing next to me, is all I can bring myself to remember. I think that's how it happened. I am already tipsy. Then he speaks to me above the infinite, ear-thumping music. I'm deafened by the racket. I pretend to listen. I cannot respond, so I smile instead. We go outside for a while to wrap ourselves in the cool breeze of that September night. It's there when I actually see him, hear him. I like him from that moment on, though we play it safe and easy for a while.

We are full of exciting ideas for our future together.

I wish Mazy was like me. They say opposite poles attract but unfortunately, that will never be our case. We may tolerate each other more now, but as always, we don't see eye to eye.

Chapter 61

Sandy

Mazy, somehow, proves me wrong and despite all adversities, she graduates with an honours degree. I admit I secretly doubted whether or not Mazy would ever graduate. I certainly don't doubt her capabilities, though I know *she* does. She could well achieve a doctorate if only she believed in herself. Yet she pushes herself to the very limits of survival. I know that sounds dramatic but it's nearly always so hard to get through the impenetrable jungle that is her mind. Totally impassable. I wonder why she seeks constant reassurance when she doesn't pay heed to sound advice.

The dawn of dawns finally awakes and an exceptional moment is lived, when her name is called out to receive her well-earned degree certification. I see her step aside from the crowd of students, she hides behind. She walks apprehensively up the aisle, cloaked in black, with tasselled mortarboard, sitting somewhat defiantly on her head. I watch incredulously, with my breath held, thinking to myself that this can't be true. Surely the girl that phones long before daybreak in complete anguish, is not the person I see in front of me now.

There she is, larger than life, receiving what has been so rightfully earned. It's cost her an arm and a leg, I know. Perhaps even an eye, but she persevered and achieved it, no matter what. And this is the girl I see up on the transformed stage, a raised structure in the altar area, for it is a church, where the ceremony is held.

I observe every detail, even when the Head of the University and tutors forming the board panel, exchange a few words with her. She nods and replies politely, I imagine, for I cannot hear what is said. She returns them a smile, that illumines her face and wipes her anxiety away. I stop crossing my fingers and stop silently praying that all goes well because it has. My heart swirls in sheer pride and my emotions spiral in blessed satisfaction. I know her father and sisters feel the same way. Throughout all these years, we have been part of Mazy's battle, either directly or indirectly and now we are here to form part of her astonishing success.

The ceremony is beautiful. Lengthy yet not one bit boring. Totally rewarding. It's enhanced by its surroundings. The quaint but sophisticated church with its high steeple, towers majestically over the rooftops of the neighbouring buildings. It is close to the university, the reason undoubtedly why it's used as the venue for the graduation ceremony. The church exterior follows the same line of red brick design as the university, a Gothic style that was a popular trend of the Victorian era. The picturesque beauty that depicts the facade does not mar in any way, the glorious interior where the grandeur and splendour of a unique architecture, is synonymous with an elegance, no longer existing today.

The Head of the University dedicates an emotive speech to the students to conclude the ceremony. With meaningful words, he highlights their perseverance and draws attention to the constancy of their efforts throughout the past years, which undoubtedly, is the key to future success. The reception that follows the heart-warming ceremony, is no less impressive and held on the large university campus. There are two enormous marquees beautifully adorned with flowers, cleverly forming the university's insignia. Long tables holding a variety of appetising food and drinks are all carefully aligned from one end of each marquee to the other. The university grounds are indeed a marvellous sight. Acres and acres of land stretch out like a green carpet, meandering lazily around the university's main building. It's a pleasure just to be there and admire the spectacular views around us.

It's also a pleasure to finally be able to put a face to every name, that Mazy may have mentioned, during her time there. It's gratifying to meet lovely crowds of students and tutors, who in some way or another, got to know Mazy well. They speak highly of her. Together they pose for the 'must have' photograph, all mortarboards flying in the air.

I wonder deep down what they must really think of her. She never disclosed her 'secret' to anyone, apparently. Those closer to her must have undoubtedly, guessed. Others? Well, who cares? Today is not a day for worries!

Chapter 62

Mazy

I'm offered a job as a lecturer at a university in Merseyside, not far from where I study. I could go for it, after all, it's a great opportunity. They don't offer it to anyone. They offer it to me. My life could change for better or worse, who knows? All I know is that I turn it down, without much thought. An erroneous decision, perhaps. I suppose I get cold feet! The thought of suddenly having my life planned out for me, gives me the jitters. I am not sure what I want or where I want to head. I don't even know if I want to continue studying or call it a day, here and now.

The only two things that really move me are my passion for music and travel. I must head in that direction, I know. If I don't try it, I will always regret it. Attempt is better than regret, I guess. Besides, I have nothing to lose, but something impedes me, as always, from taking the plunge. Something called a mind full of dim-witted monstrosities, totally senseless, yet they govern my every move.

I head for home, in the end. Perhaps another wrong move. I don't even try to seek advice as to which way to go. Nope! I just bottle it all up and continue feeling lost. Now it's even worse than before because I don't want to go back to my 'cage'. I've known freedom. At least, some kind of it. The type that I don't have to answer to anyone, not if I don't want to. Now I don't even know how to kickstart another life for me. Where do I go? How do I begin? My mind is nebulous, even more than usual.

I know I drive my family crazy with my unresponsive attitude. They don't understand my indifference. I just want to shake them off my back. That's why I want to live alone, like a hermit. They want to see me with consistent motivation, not the kind that comes in dribs and drabs. They want to see me with a secure job and a dynamic social life. Everything that is fulfilling enough for me to lead a reasonably good life, but that is not in my plans right now, because all I want to do at this present time, is think. Think and reflect on my future. Is that so hard to understand? Don't they realise that my mind is exclusive? There's certainly no match for it.

I have massive arguments with Ella, during this time. Of course, this is nothing new. Whenever we are together, the tension soars, temperatures rise, volcanoes erupt and black triumphs over white or vice versa. Anything, however minimal, for the sake of arguing. The yin and yang inside of us explode like a fused electrical connection.

It takes me three years to get my act together. During this time, I do nothing. Just live like a zombie. I sleep all day. It's so much easier to do. I don't have to talk, then. Not to anyone. I get up at night, grab a bite to eat and sit on the sofa. I stay up all night, just me and my thoughts. Some are often positive and urge me to continue in whichever way possible. A gratifying shot of optimism sweeps hysterically through all of my blood vessels and all I want to do is pack my bags and flee for the unexpected. For a future of unknown surprises, totally new surroundings and new beginnings.

In my head, I plan all the steps I'm going to take. And suddenly, I am clear as to my direction. I take the pan by the handle and feel I am in command. But, all too soon, other thoughts invade that fine line of enthusiasm and cross over into obscurity, where they become horrifically demonic. They leave me crushed, as if a towering crane or a colossal rock has descended on me with unrestrained force, converting me to stone, then crumbling me to sand. When dawn awakes, I retire to my bedroom and sleep with no notion of time, for my brain is fatigued. One vicious circle I get myself into and can't seem to break away from.

Me, myself and I...and my fearful mind.

I disclose my plans to Freya. I confide in her. Always have done, so I grant her the privilege of being the first to know. She urges me to speak to the family about my future, if only to keep them quiet for a while, or to give them some hope that I have a rekindling spirit, still within me. She's right, I know, but I am reluctant to do so. I realise they are always sceptical, though they will try their utmost not to show it. I believe they play along with me to avoid arguments. So as not to discourage me. I guess they fear that I may lose myself further and deeper into the labyrinth of depression.

They are on a high with hope when I give them a taste of what's on my plate for the future. They automatically encourage me to leave, expressing wise words of advice for my happiness. I'm glad they support my decision and although I don't want to sound negative, I wonder if, at this point, they are relieved that they will get rid of me soon. Perhaps they are just being cautious, mouthing the right words, so as not to destroy the little motivation that surprisingly, I let bubble to the surface, from time to time.

Chapter 63

Sandy

You probably know Mazy by now, if you have read this far! We know she doesn't make things simple for herself. The countless restrictions and limitations that she purposely imposes on herself, are beyond all logical conception and certainly mind-blowing for those around her. She confirms she's on a mission now. I believe her. The family believes her, even though *she* may doubt it. We are pleased. Who wouldn't be? I'm just thankful for any progress she makes, for any minuscule step along the way, for she is unique.

We speak and she agrees that before she can act, her mind has to be crystal clear about how she is going to dispose of her precious belongings. She cannot take everything with her, otherwise, she would. I admit she cannot get up one morning and start to empty her wardrobe, cupboards and drawers and tell herself, this I will keep and this I will give away. It definitely doesn't work like that with her, so she sets herself deadlines which, deep down, she knows are unrealistic. Consequently, she repeatedly sets herself new milestones, which continue to be unachievable, given the amount of stuff she has accumulated through the years. Stuff that she has never used and I'm sure, she never will. Stuff which, I doubt, she remembers hoarding since childhood. Though her photographic memory, which boasts a special place in her mind, proves us wrong. It has shot to absolute perfection every microscopic detail. Therefore, all is safely lodged in her brain to her complete satisfaction. That omnipotent mind will not forget anything, however trivial and insignificant.

She is fully aware of where everything stands, sits, hangs, or hides. No corner escapes her. No nook or cranny is left without being searched or emptied. Everything is scanned and scrutinised till Mazy's eyes almost fall out of their sockets, in total exhaustion.

It takes three long years, with its thirty-six months or one hundred and fifty-six weeks, for Mazy to sort everything out and hopefully, even herself. During this time, there are many moments in which she falls into utter desperation and doubts whether or not she will ever pack her bags and go. We can't help but doubt it ourselves, though we make endless efforts to encourage her along the way. We try our hardest to disguise how we truly feel, for we fear at times and even often, that she will never take off.

So, alongside Mazy's mind, my mind too, is a tidal wave of commotion. Will she stay, will she leave, will she not? If she goes, where will she live, where will she work? What will she do when she gets down? Who will she turn to? Then, I snap out of it, as I always do. She's been alone at university, hasn't she? She knows now how to fend for herself. She's no fool. Of course, she can stand on her own two feet and move forward. Nothing to worry about, or to panic. Besides, her family is only a phone call away, no matter how far she goes. She's not the only person in the world, diagnosed with OCD or Pure O, or whatever it is they call it. She will manage, no matter what it takes.

And we continue with our lives in wait of what the future may bring, often in unavoidable apprehension, as we can never ascertain anything, assume or even guess when it comes to Mazy.

Chapter 64

Mazy

I have to start somewhere, though. So, I decide to go through all the books, documents, paperwork and even receipts that no one needs, but are hoarded nevertheless, from heaven knows when. I realise now I am a hoarder, too. Something I never realised until now. It suddenly dawned on me that I am a stasher, and *that* makes me really nervous. I've seen so many documentaries about people who hoard without notion or control, till they have barely room to move about in their homes. Thankfully, I'm not that bad. But if I continue saving whatever is useless, I will undoubtedly fit the bill. Make it to that category.

With each gnawing ache that travels through every recess, there could be in both my body and mind, I set out, incredulously, to achieve the most complicated task I feel I've ever had to do, part with my worldly possessions. Touch them, take them out of their sacred places. Can't anybody understand that that for me it's synonymous with a felony, even blasphemy, profanity? Dramatic perhaps, but not for me. For me, it's a sacrilege.

My blessed belongings! For so long unscathed. Presently heading for the trash, or to someone else's hands, who will not take the same care of them as I did. It's so hard a step to take, especially when nobody understands. People would scorn me if they could see me and I shudder in shameful apprehension.

Totally unheard of, unseen, until now. That is what my family must be thinking, whilst witnessing something they never dreamed could possibly happen one day. I even astonish myself. Things that have been buried away for years, (I can even call them *things* now) are actually in my hands, whilst I toy with the idea if I should give them away or simply bin them! I would have been absolutely traumatised if I had thought about doing this, years or even months ago.

There is suddenly this arduous, often gruelling sensation, slowly spreading inside me and compelling me to continue. Forcing me not to give up. It must be how badly I want to move on, to start a new life, without looking back. But as much as I want to hurry along and get everything sorted, I'm often paralysed or stuck to the ground. Brain dead. Immobile. Depleted of adrenaline and energy. And I wrestle desperately with my inner self, for this time, I must conquer my endless war. I *really* must keep going.

I need a focus, some kind of beacon that will guide me to my future. I cannot stay here. Lost. Completely. Without a goal or determination. It's impossible to live when I feel dead. I don't know if I will feel the same way, when I return to England. It scares me to think that. I panic and fret and I remain frozen, yet again.

No! Quickly! I can't give up and I *won't*. There are millions of things I still have to sort out. I must do away with this, that and the other. Hundreds of this, that and the other. By the time I finish, there'll be thousands. I'll breathe placidly when all is done. I'll keep my composure, though I want to scream to the universe,

Susan Cabezutto

"WHY AM I LIKE THIS?"

Chapter 65

Freya

Mazy finally buys the plane ticket and has a date for her departure. The 31st August 2017. Impressive. Couldn't have imagined it, if I tried. Not with all the turmoil that has controlled Mazy's life, for as far back as I can recall.

"Where there's a will, there's a way!" I proudly advise her. She's made me proud, alright. I think this is the best decision she can take and I can't wait for her to have a life of her own. Whether it's near or far, who cares? As long as she is happy with goals and ambitions for her to achieve, I know she'll make it.

I ask her if it's been worth it. All that hardship and constant worries that have engulfed and constricted her senses throughout her younger years, regarding her room and her forever prized belongings. Has it all been worth her while?

The continuous rituals, like harrowing torture inflicted on herself by herself. The excruciating fears that dampness would invade her sanctuary, bleed through the walls, like an evil spirit and creep into the furniture, ruining her priceless belongings. Then again, robbers could steal them or a massive fire could make them disintegrate in a fraction of a second. With one blink of an eye, everything could vanish into thin air. Your sanctuary and your precious stuff!

And now, look at you! The irony of it all! You have spent three years discarding or giving away every single one of those stupid, absolutely, stupid stuff, that you so obsessively treasured or buried in your room. Not once did you enjoy them because you never knew how. You never listened to any of us, whilst you built an empire of anxiety and distress that was so unrealistic. But you couldn't come to terms with that, could you? And all for nothing, because soon you'll be on your way to a whole new life, with just yourself. Everything else will be left behind. Just like when you die.

I wonder if Mazy takes it all in. I wonder if this three-year exercise is an eye-opener for her. It must be. Surely, she must be thinking how foolish she has been to give her utmost priority, throughout her life, to what is totally insignificant.

I suppose, the time she spent just looking lost and lifeless to her family, which were days on end, she was actually reflecting on her future. I sincerely hope that in this future there is no time for obsessions. No stumbling with the same stone all over again or falling into the same trap, no matter where she is or what she does.

She's older now too. More experienced. Surely, she must realise her mistakes and try to make amends. For her sake and that of her family, who have always been by her side in her best and worst moments. It's only fair, I should think, for her to turn over the page and start a whole, new chapter in her life. A clean slate. That's what we are all anxiously waiting for, without trying to make her feel overwhelmed. This family couldn't have been more patient with her.

So learn the lesson, Mazy! Because nothing is *that* valuable that you have to become obsessive about. Not even people, let alone material things. You can, for once, start over with just yourself. It takes nothing more or nothing less.

Chapter 66

Ella

I don't think anyone can be more pleased than I to see Mazy start a new life away from us. I know this doesn't sound very humane, so don't get me wrong. We are adults now and the past is the past. We move on without any grudges, after all, we are siblings and blood is thicker. Isn't it? Or so they say.

I've always said that Mazy must stand on her own two feet. Have no one to rely on but herself. That's probably the only way she will ever come to terms with that radical mind of hers. And *finally*, she takes the greatest dive into the deep end, we could ever have imagined. I must admit I'm really proud of her. I always doubted she'd make this grand move. But she already proved me wrong, once - when she went to university. I never expected her to go, or even to finish her degree. I always thought she'd return home one day, looking lost and forlorn. But she didn't. Instead, she came back with a B Sc (Hons) title after her name. Admirable, I must say. I realise now, how hard it must have been for her. I for one, wouldn't have been able to persevere. I know how quickly I would have given up.

Now the best thing she can do is to start afresh. A new place to live, new job, new people to meet, new friends to make and new entertainment to enjoy. I really hope she goes dressed from head to toe with a positive attitude. Leaving right behind her, all those negative vibes that have enveloped her since childhood. There's no room in life for negativity. It's harmful to one's body and mind. It makes you feel small and withdrawn and doesn't allow you to blossom or progress. It plummets your self-esteem to the very pits of the earth until all there is left to do is barely breathe, because even breathing is repressive.

She must find happiness, too. In whichever way, shape or form. Happiness in the shape of a person, a friend or simply having peace of mind. Happiness is by far, the most important thing in life. Next to good health, of course! This is the only way to live. Not in fear, not in distress, just in sheer contentment. Until that is achieved, I know she can't be happy in life.

I realise no one takes me seriously. They think I'm the world's greatest scatterbrain. Nobody thinks I'm capable of having some organised thoughts in my mind. But believe you and me, my mind is absolutely crammed with organised thoughts that make me the most positive, encouraging and happiest person that ever there was. At least, I know where I'm heading and what it is I want in this life.

There may be obstacles in the way but I don't care. I either jump over them, if in a hurry or walk cautiously around them at a slower time. But I overcome them, somehow, because I know how to play my cards, alright. I know what my priorities are too and I do not waste time. I grab the opportunities that come my way, so I never lose the train, as I sit on the right wagon, nearly always.

So there, Mazy! That's some sound advice from the sister you never got on with. I admit I never really made it easy for you, but despite our many differences, I wish you every success in your new, exciting adventure. Believe in yourself, Mazy and you'll always be a winner.

Chapter 67

Mazy

When London meets girl, it realises how very lost she is. She's definitely in the right place then! There are millions of lost souls in this city, from all walks of life, craving desperately for a better life, a quest for adventure or simply an impulsive change. I suppose it isn't much different to any other place where you may happen to start anew.

London is heaving. Everyone is here, or so it seems, hustling and bustling their lives away. Being moved or shoved around to their destiny. I'd like to see them from a bird's eye view. Scurrying dots on the ground, like ants to their nests, ready to comply with their queen's wishes. It's absolutely chaotic, but I knew *that* already. I experienced this havoc when I left for university and it's no different now. Definitely no different to the pandemonium that is in my mind, racketing through my brain, till my senses are on the verge of an outburst.

I probably won't stay here for long. I'll be on the move as soon as my pockets are full. I'll tour the world with my songs, with my own compositions. I'll continue where I left off and resume those musical skills that are currently dormant. It's what keeps me gunning my engines, till one day, they are revved up to full power. And, willing and able, I shall take off, never to be stopped.

A step at a time, though. I return to the present for today is today and it is still not over. I think back. It was hard to part from the family, even Ella and that's saying something! But I'm glad I did it. If I hadn't taken the plunge, I would probably still be alternating the sofa for the bed, all day long. Thinking, scheming and dreaming but never making it happen. My dead self with my dead life.

Hardest of all was saying bye to Mum. After all, she has been the strongest of pillars in this haphazard life of mine and still is, no matter the miles we share between us. I caught her pushing back the tears, under a cool exterior. I could tell she was anguished. Her face was falling through, when parting finally became a crude reality for all of us. I had been just as dubious of this moment, as everyone else. But it ultimately arrived. Like everything in my life, it comes in a rather random and chaotic way. Nobody expects me to take action; they are so used to seeing me 'paralysed' for so long. Somehow, I manage to do it eventually.

Mum kept eying me intently, as if my image would be erased from her mind, the moment I disappeared. I don't really know what was going through her head, in all honesty. A mixture of bitter-sweet emotions, no doubt. She said she was taking in the attractive, young woman I had become who stood there in front of her, arms clad with bags, guitar on back and a plane to catch.

"This is it, Mum, I'm never coming back, at least, not in a long time," I vowed fervently, also trying hard to fight the tears and most of all, the memories. Memories of struggle, of hardship, of a lost childhood. Even lost teens.

We all hugged as one when the flight was announced for the last time. Speechless. Knotted throats. There were so many words we wanted to say to each other. But I guess, we had both gone over this moment too many times and words are actually unnecessary. Actions and even eyes speak louder, for they have a voice of their own. Besides, I just wanted to flee and start afresh, in search of a new life that I so badly deserved to live.

Without a blink, they held their gaze fixed on me, as the escalator slowly carried me up to board my flight. We waved energetically until I finally vanished out of sight. Then those tears we had tried so hard to suppress, now gushed unrestrained. I hastily tried to hide them behind the dark sunglasses, sitting idly on the top of my head.

I sat by the window, in the hope I could still catch a glimpse of that wonderful family, to whom I hadn't often shown much gratitude. When the plane roared off, with engines revving explosively as it soared, I realised Mum had whispered something in my ear. Broken words, almost inaudible.

"Don't let the demons in your mind win, Mazy. Never give up and don't ever look back."

I guess that's what I've always tried to do, Mum. Ever since I can remember, I have always tried desperately *not* to give up. Hopefully, I never will.

Chapter 68

Mazy

The hotel throws me a warm, inviting look and is there, waiting for me to alight from a taxi I was lucky to catch. Most of them were darting dangerously, yet skilfully, in and out of ongoing traffic, as if it were their last day on earth. It's busier around the city centre, I imagine, and it's summer, too. The hotel exterior seems rather grungy, almost decrepit at first sight. Just like my mood, tumbling, like always. I was told it was decent but I shall reserve my opinion until I see the interior. The exterior could certainly do with an uplift.

My heart sinks from one minute to the other. The excitement suddenly seems to deflate. Maybe reality kicks in. The reality of knowing that this is it. After years of dreaming and scheming and disciplining my mind for the move, I find myself in my new 'home' alone and far away from the faces I've always known. I'm becoming dramatic now, I know.

Snap out of it, girl! Get your act together, once and for all! About time, too. Do you want to be stuck in a rut for the rest of your life?

This is the good side of my mind speaking, not where the demons dwell. The side that encourages me to continue my quest with whatever strength and dignity remains. The side that beseeches, almost plaintively and always in sheer desperation, for me not to give up. I can't help feeling scared. There's no turning back now. I *have* to make this work for me. So many hidden emotions that I've tried hard to bury, surface unremorsefully. It tightens my throat, till I can no longer breathe. Again, the bitter taste of bile stings sharply, as if I've swallowed a bunch of nettles or thistles. And this is just the beginning. I have a strong feeling in my bones, that the first year of adaptation will be the worst. If I can overcome this, I am sure that I can overcome (well, if not overcome, perhaps better control) my disorder. I say this with conviction.

The hotel waits. OK. In we go. I sigh hesitantly. My heartbeat fails. I cannot sink in quicksand. Not right now, anyway. I must stay calm and positive. My mind must not be swimming in mud and sludge. I step inside, heaving my luggage up the beaten access ramp.

At last, I am pleasantly surprised. True enough, the hotel seems pretty decent, once inside. At least what I can observe from the foyer seems 'acceptable'. I quickly scan everything around me. An eco-friendly theme reigns throughout. Evergreens fuse perfectly with eye-catching potpourris of pink and white-petalled amaryllises. They are expertly assembled in stylish copper pots, that notch up a sense of grandeur no terracotta pot ever would. Even soft, silky tulips in peach shades, are expertly nestled in the array. They dangle audaciously from ceiling corners that stand out prominently against pastel-coloured walls or rest majestically at the sides of the antique, French-styled reception counter.

Most captivating of all are the ceiling murals with their vintage hand-crafted, exclusive designs. Maybe old English or Italian, I cannot quite make up my mind. But they are absolutely stunning and the greenery blends to perfection, without shunning their glory.

I look away reluctantly, as they provide the calming embrace I needed and catch the receptionist, waiting for me.

"Everyone marvels at the sight, particularly as the hotel exterior is disappointing and requires urgent refurbishment. It will be taken care of soon. Clients must be kept satisfied at all costs," she smiles. No need to complain now.

I check in quickly and move to the fourth floor where my feet almost sink into the thick, tweed-patterned carpets that deeply line the snaked corridors, so I tug at the wheels of my luggage, lest they refuse to move.

I plonk myself heavily on the bed. The room is light and airy, almost clinical. A neutral decor prevails. It's something I welcome. The 'less is more' effect on rooms works better for my mind. I don't have to take in so much at once; the checking rituals become easier. I hope.

Pictures of carefree landscapes, replicating a Van Gogh style, catch my eye. Maybe because I am an art lover or maybe because they are so perfectly aligned. They are, indeed, a focal point. To my right, blue, fly away curtains drape the windows. Not bad at all. I am pleasantly relieved. The off-white marbled ensuite bathroom isn't displeasing either. It's impeccable. I have what I need. I can't really ask for more.

I want to relax now but I am not allowed to do so. *Never* allowed, somehow. Sheer panic rapidly swarms my thoughts. It oppresses my every limb, and demons possess me, once again.

The realisation that I only have four days to find somewhere cheap to stay seizes my will and makes me hyperventilate.

I knew it wasn't going to be easy. Nothing cheap will be safe, naturally. I should have found somewhere decent to stay before I left home. But then, I had a crap mobile phone at the time, from where I could research absolutely nothing. I would have had to search for rental properties on my laptop, only to get caught in sorting three years of accumulated emails. And I did so want to move on!

Chapter 69

Sandy

The pandemic creeps unexpectedly upon us, like the demons in Mazy's mind, that spread and mutate through her brain, so very aware of her vulnerability. Likewise, this wretched virus, which we keep hearing about in every media on earth, is swarming hastily through every country, eclipsing everyone into vague darkness and shadows. Leaving its mark on whoever it preys on. And with it, my fears for Mazy increase three-fold. How will she cope now? She has lived all her life with the anguish of catching germs and her hand-washing rituals are excruciating and mortifying. She'll be dying inside, I'm sure. I know she has always lived in lockdown. But right now, it's a lockdown by law, not by forced will and that can't be an easy ride for her, either.

She has been doing so well for herself, I am told. Mastering those wretched rituals as best as she can and gradually, overcoming many of the restrictions and limitations, she has always created for herself. It makes me feel so impotent, even angry that all this is happening. It's absolutely incredible. Such bad timing, too! I so wish that it doesn't make Mazy retreat, yet again, into that bottomless pit, from where she has been trying so desperately to emerge, all her life.

Ever since she arrived, she's tried to overcome the obstacles in her way, with great determination. I think I've lost count of the many times she's fallen and picked herself up again. Good on you, girl! As long as you keep trying and moving forward, I can breathe calmly and even keep my composure. Your family can too.

Mazy searches for a place to stay, as a priority. She could extend her stay in the hotel if need be, but knowing Mazy, she will not rest until she has a place of her own. So, she didn't really have much choice but to look for something sooner rather than later. She searches tirelessly online and visits most of the places she believes could be safe and worth their price.

Camden is among those places that enthral her. Maybe because of the pulsating life that seems to emanate from that town. Everything that Mazy compels herself to miss. But, *hopefully*, not any more. She tells me she takes the subway and confesses feeling like the 'Girl on the Train' sitting there, staring out of the window. Obviously, with a different purpose but still staring out into the unknown; a 'drunken' mind, catching a glimpse of houses, landscapes and people, that are subsequently gone forever. Then, submerging back into the zigzagging maze of underground tunnels, where the darkness is so absolutely blinding.

Camden meets her expectations. It is the place for her. She knows right in her head and heart that this is where she wants to live and make it. It's *so* cool. So colourful. It makes her feel good. She roams the place, more animatedly than ever before, as she takes in the vibrancy, the vitality, the energy, the youthfulness. Even the joie de vivre, something Mazy hasn't felt in her lifetime. She describes everything so vividly, it so pleases me to hear.

The shops are jam-packed with stuff she's always fancied. Shoes, bags, the black, rock gear she's been after for ages. So much variation, it would be impossible to choose. She's swept off her feet, I know.

Music of all genres blares contemptuously from every corner. No one complains. So, it continues to boom intrepidly, almost heroically. People stride along aimlessly to the beat. Some break-dance on the overly trodden pavement. Crowds gather, clapping wildly, ready to join in. They have no cares in the world. They are free and happy. Will Mazy be like that one day? It's my only wish.

The enticing smells of mouth-watering food from the food markets radiate such magnetism, that readily allure the passers-by. Each stall is more deliciously appetising than the previous one. There's something here for everyone's taste, I believe. But the money, I wonder if there's something here to fit everyone's pocket?

Nevertheless Mazy is here for one purpose, so she needs to step down from cloud nine, or wherever she's enwrapped and move fast. She vows to herself she must return - *definitely*. She studies her map, comparing it to the one on her mobile. Camden cannot be tackled in a day, evidently. The many estate agents she talks to on the prospects of renting, all share a common conviction, despite their art of persuasion.

Their first question is the expected 'What's your annual income?' When they realise Mazy has still to look for a job, they tell her to return when she has it. It is that simple. Nothing comes out of nothing. No money, no doors open. She can't be thinking properly if she thought she could find something suitable and affordable there and then. We must be practical and reasonable and be open to the reality of things.

But what Mazy can be assured of, is that one day, she will live in the best apartment she can afford there or anywhere. Her mystical intuition and those deep-rooted, innate feelings in her heart, will prove her right, somehow. It keeps her from falling into despair, as now there are only three days left before she has a roof over her head. Or is it two?

Exhausted and thwarted but still positive, Mazy heads back into the subway, hotel bound.

Epilogue

Mazy

Five years on, almost six! It's uncanny how time flies. I'm settled in North London, living in single adult accommodation. It suits me just fine for now until I can afford to buy a place of my own, and that will be sooner rather than later.

I've gone from being a barista at Starbucks to a postal manager, taking a break from psychology. But not for long, for I have returned to my roots and I currently work as a psychologist, alternating this with being a lecturer at a local university. Experience in anything and everything is the mother of success. It wasn't an easy venture and still isn't, but music helps to see me through my dark days.

I sing in pubs most weekends, on open mike nights. People like me. They stop to listen, just like at university. They even like my own compositions. I'm getting quite well-known around this area and it looks more like five days have gone by rather than five years.

I've lived through many things already, even a pandemic, just like everyone else on this planet. Something that wasn't foreseen and sprung upon us, with little warning. I only had *myself* to rely on. *Me*, to sort myself out. *Me,* to run my own life. *Me*, just me.

These were strange times and they still are. I laughed in people's faces. It's not like me to do so, but I just wanted to shout to the world:

"Now you know what it feels to be condemned to the fear of catching viruses and germs. Of constant hand washing with antiseptics, until the skin is as dried as a prune, or as tight as the stretched membrane, that enfolds a cavernous drum."

In fact, I don't feel scared anymore, for I see I am not alone. The whole world lives in fear and is immersed in rituals, they never even dreamed they would, one day, fall into.

It's all very weird. Whereas people feel insecure and apprehensive, I seem to have lost most of my insecurities, for I know better than most, how it feels to be obsessive against your will. I have always lived like that.

I observe neighbours, friends and colleagues. They do not realise how frantic a person can suddenly become, entangled helplessly in a supreme mania that turns their whole world upside down. The changes they can instantaneously go through, without notion or logic. The robotic actions they had no clue they could systematically enact. Even without coherence. Now they do.

I watch them, practically daily, delve into their pockets for forgotten masks and panic at the thought of having their faces undressed. Naked. Unwillingly inviting in this terrifying bug that is suddenly top-ranked globally, as the most lethal illness ever to be imagined. I can't believe that everything else now takes a second place if no place at all.

They sanitise and decontaminate like there's no tomorrow. From bags to groceries, from counters to kitchen worktops and bathrooms to floors, everything must be totally immaculate. Every nook and cranny, whether personal or public must be flawless.

The soles on shoes are manically sterilised with antibacterial sprays, which no one ever gave a thought to before. They are left outside, their entrance forbidden. Clothes are stripped off. Straight to the wash. Bleach is back in full force. Its unbearable smell which travels painfully through nostrils, seems not to be obnoxious anymore.

No one can touch. NO! Hands have been warned. Fingers prohibited. Banned. Knuckles take over. Elbows now speak for some. "Hi! How are you?" They greet hesitantly. Bannisters, escalators, elevator call buttons and door knobs are the enemy. Beware! Nobody wants a visit from this invincible microbe. Do they?

The worse thing of all is that once your mind becomes obsessive, the rituals flourish and harvest in abundance. They take over. Without barely any coherent awareness, you are enslaved. As if you have sold your soul to the devil or the most powerful of mafias around.

You are not *you* anymore. You are what your mind wants you to be. It hurls you into a deplorable, loathsome state that takes a lifetime and beyond to master and defeat. A daily battle. Otherwise, you are consumed and callously devoured, till there is not a drop of energy left in you. Only asphyxia.

No one can believe how living alone can actually help. How keeping busy can counteract the most persistent of thoughts or voices that echo heartlessly through a brain on fire. *No one*. Nor how this recent pandemic has given me the confidence to grow and help others, for I shall dedicate most of my time to decipher the mind, to decode the most encrypted of messages, that can give us light at the end of the tunnel. But most importantly, the realisation that I am really not alone, gives me the peace of mind I've always yearned for. I am not that rare, unique, alien I thought I was. Because anybody can become neurotic, at any given time in their lives. From one sad day to the next.

So, let's hang on in there those of you, who like me, are lost in that maze of a mind; who are held hostage against your will. Let's persevere in our endeavour to win. And it doesn't matter how many bad days still lurk ahead that make us fall, for after each fall, we shall pick ourselves up to face a better day.

It is the most difficult mission that life has thrust upon us. But with every little grain of support that we can give each other, we *will* survive. If anything, to tell the tale of how, eventually, we managed to defeat Goliath and all the Goliaths that may dwell in our ever so powerful, intricate minds.

An Ode to An Amazing Person

Where do I start to describe,
A person so full of conviction and strive.
From the day you were born no doubt,
When both the sun and the stars were about,
To mark a beginning so wondrous and great,
Of one so oblivious to her forthcoming fate.
The heavens, in its generosity,
Loaned its best soul
To live 'neath the body of a baby whose goal,
Had still to be written for her future role.
From the very first moment your eyes met mine,
I knew there was something sincere and divine.
That look in those eyes
So piercing, so vivid, so pure, so refined,
For a baby whose very sole purpose on earth,
Was set to commence from the instant of birth.
The wheel of fortune had slowly been spun,
By a hand from above who conjured a plan,
And firmly believed that you'd be the one,
To attain all those triumphs that lay well ahead,
In that marvellous future that awaits to be led,
By someone so special, so ingenious,
So incredibly grand,
Blessed with a mind only one of its brand.
A mind so prodigious and so remarkably powerful,
Yet so very docile and exquisitely wonderful.

In Defeat of Goliath

A mind you control more and more each day,
With the might and the strength you have hidden away.
So unlock your kind heart – throw away the key,
And start paving the way for your destiny.
Spread out your wings and fly high like a bird,
Sing out to the world, let your voice be heard.
Send your message of love, hope and faith to unite,
Each and every one fighting in defeat of their plight,
And believe me, my dearest, as I do know at length,
That you shall accomplish with unbelievable strength,
Your goals and your dreams, all dormant since childhood.
So remember these words when depressed is your mood.
Because every good thing that occurs in this world
Will be down to your marvellous, so distinctive a voice,
That projects such amazing songs for all to rejoice.

Acknowledgements

My most sincere gratitude to my family for their constant encouragement and for always believing in me.

A special, most heartfelt thank you to my publishers, Michael Terence Publishing (MTP), especially to a marvellous team, Keith Abbott (Executive Director), Caroline Mylon (Editor) and Karolina Robinson Zammit (Creative Executive Director) for your guidance and professionalism, and for giving me this wonderful opportunity to relay my story to the whole wide world. You have helped me achieve a childhood dream. So thank you from the bottom of my heart.

*Available worldwide from Amazon
and all good bookstores*

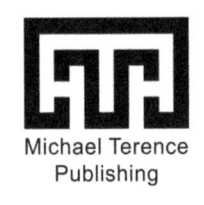

Michael Terence
Publishing

www.mtp.agency

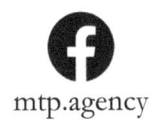

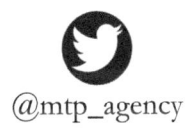

mtp.agency

@mtp_agency

Milton Keynes UK
Ingram Content Group UK Ltd.
UKHW021618030823
426158UK00010B/28

9 781800 945944